Consciousness, awareness and pain in general anaesthesia

Consciousness, awareness and pain in general anaesthesia

Edited by

M. Rosen MB, ChB, FFARCS
Honorary Professor in Anaesthetics,
University Hospital of Wales, Cardiff

J. N. Lunn MD, FFARCS
Reader in Anaesthetics,
University of Wales College of Medicine, Cardiff

Butterworths
London Boston Durban Singapore Sydney Toronto Wellington

First published, 1987

© **Butterworth & Co. (Publishers) Ltd, 1987**

British Library Cataloguing in Publication Data

Consciousness, awareness and pain in general anaesthesia
   1. Anaesthesia
   I. Rosen, M. (Michael)   II. Lunn, John N.
   617'.96   RD81

   ISBN 0-407-00749-0

Library of Congress Cataloging in Publication Data

Consciousness, awareness, and pain in general anaesthesia

   Includes bibliographies and index.
   1. Anesthetics—Physiological effect.
2. Consciousness. 3. Awareness. 4. Pain. I. Rosen,
Michael. II. Lunn, John N. [DNLM: 1. Anesthesia,
General. 2. Cognition. 3. Consciousness. WO 275 C755]
RD82.C66   1987   615'.781   87-23871
ISBN 0-407-00749-0

Photoset by Butterworths Litho Preparation Department
Printed and bound in Great Britain by Anchor Brendon Ltd,
Tiptree, Essex

Introduction

A patient who has general anaesthesia expects oblivion, is horrified by the prospect of becoming awake unexpectedly, and is terrified of 'talking' inappropriately. One could, at first, easily and confidently reassure them that general anaesthesia 20 years ago would guarantee unconsciousness. However, this certainty became somewhat dented when a report appeared of recall during surgery with the aid of hypnosis, even with apparently properly administered general anaesthesia and spontaneous ventilation. All this was easily – or fairly easily – put aside as a curiosity with expressions of concern about the 'apparently' and 'properly administered' nature of the anaesthesia, or the lack of objectivity in the hypnotic analysis. But many anaesthetists were uneasy; some applied earplugs, others serenaded the patients with euphonious and encouraging choruses. More recent work has reopened the question, and indeed supported the earlier findings.

The introduction of muscle relaxants made it possible for patients to be kept immobile while conscious. The advantages of light anaesthesia for major surgery became apparent, with much less circulatory depression, so it was adopted. However, the signs of anaesthesia were blurred, sometimes to extinction, and a complication arose – 'awareness', sometimes accompanied by an agonizing step-by-step memory of the surgical operation. This new truly terrifying experience – even in the days before anaesthesia surgical speed somewhat mitigated the horror – soon spawned moves for compensation, or maybe revenge. The courts acted and the first case in the UK of a caesarean section received an award. Many others, and not pregnant patients only, await judgement. And the same is true in the USA.

The wider use of analgesic drugs, which even in large doses may not guarantee unconsciousness, has produced the sentient, but pain-free patient, who may complain of unanticipated awareness.

The whole field called out for consideration by a master class. A two-day workshop was therefore arranged in Cardiff in June 1986 attended by anaesthetists, neurophysiologists, psychologists, legal and medicolegal experts from both sides of the Atlantic. This book is *not* an account of these proceedings, but the writers were chosen mainly from the participants, and their chapters are enhanced by presentations and discussions at the workshop. Much was learnt, including how much more should be done to elucidate, to manage and to prevent these problems. There are in this book, therefore, the seeds for future research, but there is also practical advice for the clinician struggling to cope with these unhappy complications. Perhaps, the expectation of the patient for oblivion on every occcasion cannot easily, or ever, be met. However, anaesthetist readers will now certainly do better, lawyers will be well informed, and neurophysiologists and psychologists can see new fields for their activities and investigations. Some patients will have much for which to thank the contributors.

Michael Rosen

v

Acknowledgements

The workshop on which this book is based was sponsored by the following firms and it is a pleasure to acknowledge their help:

Imperial Chemical Industries Pharmaceuticals
Janssen Pharmaceuticals
Roche Products
Anaquest
Ohmeda
Datex Instrumentarium
S.L.E.
Cadwell Europe
Medical Defence Union
The Wellcome Trust
Antec Systems

Contributors

H. L. Bennett PhD
Department of Anesthesiology, University of California, Davis Medical Center, Sacramento, California, USA

L. J. Couture BA
Research Technologist II, Department of Anesthesiology, University of Louisville, Louisville, Kentucky, USA

R. C. Dutton MD
Department of Anesthesiology, Kaiser Permanente Medical Center, Hayward, California, USA

H. L. Edmonds Jr PhD
Professor and Director of Research, Department of Anesthesiology, University of Louisville, Louisville, Kentucky, USA

J. M. Evans MB, BCh, FFARCS
Consultant Anaesthetist, Nuffield Department of Anaesthetics, The Radcliffe Infirmary, Oxford, UK

M. Frank MB, ChB, DA, FFARCS
Senior Lecturer and Honorary Consultant, Anaesthetic Unit, The London Hospital Medical College, London, UK

L. Goldmann PhD
Child Care and Development Group, University of Cambridge, Cambridge, UK

R. L. Hargrove MB, FFARCS
Consultant Anaesthetist, Westminster Hospital, London, UK

L. Herregods MD
Staff Anaesthetist, Department of Anaesthesiology, University of Ghent University Hospital, Ghent, Belgium

J. G. Jones MD, FFARCS
Professor of Anaesthesia, Department of Anaesthesia, University of Leeds, Leeds, UK

W. W. Mapleson DSc, FInstP
Professor of the Physics of Anaesthesia, Department of Anaesthetics, University of Wales College of Medicine, Cardiff, UK

E. M. Papper MD, FFARCS (Hon)
Professor, University of Miami, Florida, USA

M. J. Powers MB BS, DA
Barrister of Lincoln's Inn and the Inner Temple, London, UK

Pamela F. Prior MD, MRCP
Consultant in charge of Clinical Neurophysiology, Department of Neurological Sciences, St Bartholomew's Hospital, London, UK

M. Puxon QC, MD, FRCOG
Queen's Counsel and Recorder, Temple, London, UK

G. Rolly MD, PhD
Professor in Anaesthesia and Head, Department of Anaesthesiology, University of Ghent University Hospital, Ghent, Belgium

H. Schwilden MD
Institute of Anaesthesiology, University of Bonn, Bonn, GFR

W. D. Smith PhD
Biomedical Engineering Program, California State University, Sacramento, California, USA

P. J. Standen PhD
Lecturer in Behavioural Sciences, Department of Psychiatry, Queens Medical Centre, Nottingham, UK

H. Stoeckel MD
Institute of Anaesthesiology, University of Bonn, Bonn, GFR

Sandra L. Stolzy MD
Assistant Professor, Department of Anesthesiology, University of Louisville, Louisville, Kentucky, USA

B. H. Thompson AB, JD, MBA
Professor, Stanford Law School, Stanford, California, USA

N. Ty Smith MD
Professor of Anesthesia, UCSD, VA Medical Center, San Diego, California, USA

J. E. Utting MB, FFARCS
Professor of Anaesthesia, The University Department of Anaesthesia, Royal Liverpool Hospital, Liverpool, UK

M. D. A. Vickers MB, FFARCS, FFARACS (Hon)
Professor of Anaesthetics, Department of Anaesthetics, University of Wales College of Medicine, Cardiff, UK

D. C. White MB, FFARCS
Department of Anaesthetics, Northwick Park Hospital and Clinical Research Centre, Harrow, UK

Contents

Chapter 1

Anaesthesia: a privation of the senses
An historical introduction and some definitions

D. C. White

There is interest in defining the term 'general anaesthesia' for a number of reasons. In modern practice the anaesthetized subject often subsists in a zone uncomfortably close to consciousness and in which certain manifestations of consciousness, for instance responsiveness, may be uncovered if observations are made in an appropriate way. Clearly the use of muscle relaxants (which, in fact, are paralysing agents) is chiefly responsible for this state of affairs, since their use blocks the motor response to surgery. Lest it should be thought that awareness is entirely a modern problem, the following is a short historical digression.

The first public demonstration of general anaesthesia was the famous event of October 16th 1846 at the Massachusetts General Hospital. The patient's name was Gilbert Abbot and the story is familiar. However, the author would like to draw attention to parts of Dr H. J. Bigelow's paper, read before the Boston Society for Medical Improvement 24 days later, describing the first anaesthetic. The operation on Gilbert Abbott was for some kind of vascular tumour of the jaw and Bigelow states: 'During the operation the patient muttered, as in a semiconscious state, and afterwards stated that the pain was considerable, though mitigated, in his own words, "as though the skin had been scratched with a hoe" '.

The second case was on the following day, October 17th, when a fatty tumour of considerable size was removed from the arm of a woman near the deltoid muscle. The account states: 'during the operation the patient betrayed occasional marks of uneasiness; but upon subsequently regaining her consciousness, professed not only to have felt no pain, but to have been insensible to surrounding objects'.

In current parlance, the first patient was a case of awareness, the second showed signs of awareness but had no subsequent recall.

To return from this digression to anaesthesia. The word was first used in its modern sense by the Greek philosopher, Dioscorides, in the first century AD when describing the narcotic effects of the plant *Mandragora*. Its use in the English language is usually ascribed to Oliver Wendell Holmes, and it was his advocacy of the word shortly after the events of October 1846, which popularized its use. It could be said that he did us a disservice in introducing a term so difficult to define. Furthermore the word 'anaesthesia', despite its respectable classical origins, does not slip easily off the tongue. Many people cannot correctly pronounce it and regrettably that includes members of our own profession. Attempts have been made to introduce other terms, the most recent being the reasoned proposal[1] to adopt the Greek word 'nothria' (torpor) but by this time 'anaesthesia' was too deeply entrenched.

Oliver Wendell Holmes considered himself to be responsible for the introduction of the word 'anaesthesia' into English, but it is to be found in use considerably earlier with reference to loss of sensation, e.g. an anaesthetic limb. An early dictionary definition is in an *Encyclopaedia Britannica* published by a Society of Gentlemen in Scotland in Edinburgh in 1771. The definition is: Anaesthesia signifies a privation of the senses[2].

Now to come at last to the point, here is an attempt at a definition of general anaesthesia:

General anaesthesia is a reversible state of depression of the central nervous system of such a degree that consciousness is lost and that on recovery nothing is recalled relating to the period of anaesthesia.

This definition starts well but gets into increasing difficulty. Take the salient points in order. *Reversibility* can be agreed to be an essential feature of anaesthesia. The next point is *depression*. Excessive stimulation and activity in the brain can, it seems, cause loss of consciousness. An example of this is a grand mal seizure. Also, a characteristic feature of the organization of even the simplest nervous system is the presence of feedback loops. Differential sensitivity to anaesthesia of portions of these loops may occur for a number of reasons. For instance, there may be more pathways, more synapses or chemical (transmitter) differences in certain parts of the loop. This may result in overall stimulation being seen for short periods in response to the anaesthetic (the stage of excitement). But anaesthetic agents do reduce and ultimately stop electrical activity in the brain, and a reduction in brain oxygen consumption during anaesthesia can now be measured[3]. It must be concluded that anaesthetic agents are correctly described as having a depressant action.

The next point in the definition concerns *consciousness*. There is difficulty in defining the word. For the present purposes it can be equated with awareness. To take it further would require involvement in many profundities. Consciousness is mind, and the relationship between brain and mind (the mind/body problem) constitutes the central problem of philosophy (*see* Chapter 2).

It is appropriate at this point to consider briefly the nature of the central nervous system, which is the seat of consciousness and target organ of our activities as anaesthetists. The brain has been strikingly described as the most complex organized structure in the universe[4]. Taylor also provided some data on its component parts. A recent estimate of the number of cells in the cerebral cortex is fourteen thousand million (14×10^9). There are 35 000 cells per mm^2 of cortical surface, each being in contact with about 600 other cells so that the number of synapses in the cortex is 10^7. Turning to the cerebellum, the number of granule cells is hard to estimate because they are so small and densely packed; one authority gives a figure of 40×10^9. The number of cells in the rest of the brain is a matter of guesswork; a total of 100×10^9 for the whole brain is a considered estimate – and each neurone is different. The combined length of all the axons is three times the distance from the earth to the moon!

The layout or wiring diagram of the brain is now being closely studied – the mapping out of the areas on the cortex onto which is projected the sensory input from, for instance, the eyes is now understood, at least in outline. The chemistry of the brain's neurotransmitters is also increasingly understood, but we are no nearer to elucidating the mechanism of consciousness. Indeed, if the interconnection of all the cells in the brain were accurately mapped, a gargantuan undertaking, it would not throw light on the genesis of consciousness.

Who or what sort of thing is in there looking at these extraordinarily complex displays of sensory information, sorting through the vast input, rejecting most items and storing others or bringing them to the highest level (consciousness) and finally pulling the levers of response? This entity is what is anaesthetized and, because it is so nebulous, there is difficulty in defining, let alone quantifying, the depression.

Quite a lot is known of the actions of anaesthetics at the cellular level, but only a little is known of their effects on parts of the central nervous system. This branch of academic anaesthesiology is frequently subsumed under the title 'mode of action of anaesthetics'. Unfortunately, even very detailed information as to how anaesthetics depress the function of nerve cells does not advance knowledge on how anaesthetics produce general anaesthesia at all. This must remain the situation until something is understood about the mechanisms of consciousness.

It has been suggested that consciousness arises in some unspecified manner when the complexity of the neural network rises above a certain level. When discussing this point in his 1976 Reith lectures on 'The mechanics of the mind', Colin Blakemore commented that few would claim that the world's combined telephone network (an undeniably enormous system of switches) had consciousness[5]. Hostility, perhaps, but consciousness surely not.

Whatever may be the truth of this, the author suggests that a monist approach has to be adopted to the mind/body problem and consciousness regarded as an attribute of the central nervous system in a similar manner to that in which luminescence is an attribute of a culture of luminous bacteria.

To return now to the definition of general anaesthesia, the final salient feature is *absence of memory* of events occurring during the period of anaesthesia. This part of the definition requires some discussion. It is now known that during general anaesthesia, incoming stimuli (or to be more precise the signals they produce) can be received and stored in the brain and never reach or be recalled to consciousness unless special measures, e.g. hypnosis, are adopted to bring this about. Alternatively, the presence of the stored data can be detected without the actual data being summoned to consciousness. The subject can be made to act in accordance with suggestions made during anaesthesia without recall of those suggestions[6].

Speech is the form of sensory input which lends itself to the study of this phenomenon, because it is an input signal that the subject can subsequently accurately reproduce from a stored memory. Alternatively, the message in the stored memory can observably influence behaviour, although the message itself cannot be recalled (a non-verbal response).

Evidence for the occurrence of phenomena of this sort during anaesthesia was first described in the well-known paper of Levinson[7] which is (perhaps misleadingly) entitled, 'States of awareness during general anaesthesia'. Ten patients, who were good subjects for hypnosis and were undergoing dental operations, were anaesthetized with thiopentone, nitrous oxide and ether. Electroencephalography (EEG) was used to assess the depth of anaesthesia and, when the EEG signal indicated a deep level (third plane, third stage), the anaesthetist stopped the operation by telling the surgeon that he was concerned about the patient's condition – 'He is blue etc.'. After a few minutes and some hyperventilation, the surgeon was told that all was well and that he could continue. One month later (the time interval may be important) the subjects were hypnotized and regressed to the actual operations. Of the 10 patients, four were able to repeat almost exactly the words used by the anaesthetist. Another four rembered hearing something, these patients becoming anxious and waking from hypnosis. The other two patients denied hearing anything.

Further evidence for the storage of spoken messages during anaesthesia is from the work of Bennett[6], in which patients anaesthetized by standard techniques received a message during the operations stating that when the speaker interviewed them post-operatively, they should pull on their ears. The occurrence and frequency of ear touching was very significantly higher in the experimental group of patients than in the control group (who had received no intra-operative message).

This and other work makes it inadequate to specify simply 'no memory' as part of the definition of anaesthesia. The available evidence suggests that deep levels of anaesthesia do not block auditory evoked responses and, if it is desired to exclude the auditory environment of the operating theatre from the patient, then blocking the pathway by occupancy –playing-in other more favourable material – may be the best solution.

The continuum of anaesthesia

An attempt will now be made to place general anaesthesia as defined above within a gradation or continuum which is shown in *Figure 1.1*. A continuum is a series of elements passing into each other. In this case the anaesthetic state is to be regarded

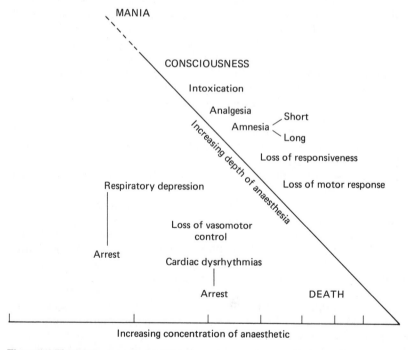

Figure 1.1 The continuum of anaesthesia

as a cumulative continuum, in that those elements whose onset indicates the higher levels of the state remain as lower levels are reached.

In *Figure 1.1*, analgesia is at the 'top' and constitutes the harbinger of anaesthesia. The word means a painless state, but it is commonly used to mean a state of reduced pain perception. This implies consciousness. Narcotic analgesics (opioids) in sufficient doses are capable of producing total analgesia or something close to it. However, they do not produce anaesthesia and this view is supported by Wong[8] in an editorial admirably entitled 'Narcotics are not expected to produce unconsciousness and amnesia'.

Nevertheless, narcotic analgesic drugs do reduce the concentration of anaesthetics needed in the brain to produce anaesthesia[9, 10]. The amount by which they do so can be fairly accurately measured by observing the depression in MAC (MAC = minimum alveolar concentration at which 50% subjects react to a specific stimulus) they produce, and there is a ceiling to this effect[11, 12]. It appears, therefore, that there is an analgesic component of anaesthesia and that pain perception is the first of the sensory modalities to be affected at the onset of the anaesthetic state.

Next in downward order comes loss of memory – amnesia – an essential component of the anaesthetic state. There is some evidence that short-term memory is affected earlier in the continuum than long-term memory. Next comes 'responsiveness'. It has been known for some time[13] that, at light levels of anaesthesia, patients may respond to spoken requests but have no memory of doing so.

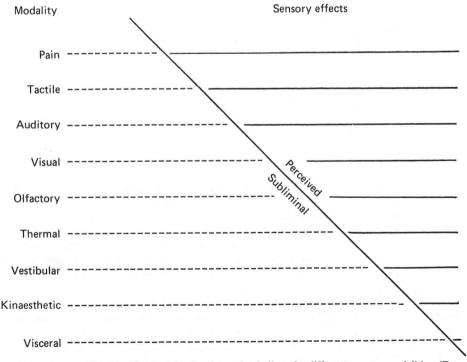

Figure 1.2 Hypothetical extents of sublimal and perceived effects for different sensory modalities. (From Dixon [14])

Continuing downwards, responsiveness is lost at the same time as perception of the other sensory modalities, and this means that, in this area, the onset of unconsciousness takes place. It may be that the different sensory modalities are not all blocked from perception at the same level of anaesthesia. *Figure 1.2* which is taken from Dixon's book *Preconscious Processing*[14] suggests that, for instance, pain stimuli may have immediate access to consciousness with little or no preconscious filtering, processing and storage, and that this results in the blunting of the perception of pain (analgesia) as one of the earliest events in the onset of the anaesthetic state. Other sensory modalities may, to a greater or lesser degree, have preconscious filtering and suppression.

The fact that responsiveness is lost at a lower level in the continuum has been known for some time. Artusio[13] showed in 1955 that, at light levels of anaesthesia, patients may respond to spoken requests but, post-operatively, have no recollection of doing so. In his experiments, intubated patients undergoing mitral valve surgery were maintained at light levels of ether/oxygen anaesthesia which was very precisely controlled and adjusted while tests were carried out to obtain the data shown in *Table 1.1*. This subject can now be studied in curarized patients, using the isolated forearm techniques.

Table 1.1 Cerebration and sensory perception during light ether/oxygen anaesthesia

	Plane 1	*Plane 2*	*Plane 3*
Amnesia	0	+++	+++
Response to voice	+++	+++	+++ → 0
Cerebration	+++	+++	+++ → 0
Recent memory	+++	+++	++ → 0
Long-term memory	+++	+++	+++ → 0
Focus of eyes	+++	+++	++ → 0
Distinguished colour	+++	+++	++ → 0
Taste	+++	+++	+++ → 0
Analgesia	0	++	+++

From Artusio[13]. Reproduced with permission, copyright 1955, American Medical Association.

At the next point in the continuum comes the loss of motor response to surgical stimulation (skin incision). This must be distinguished from the onset of generalized muscle relaxation (loss of motor tone) which occurs 'lower down' in the sequence. During the induction of anaesthesia, it is the loss of motor response to surgery which is the single most obvious and reliable sign of the onset of anaesthesia. It is a most convenient feature that the onset of unconsciousness and amnesia – two essential components of the anaesthetic state – are placed close to but above the loss of motor response in the continuum.

This is one reason for the usefulness of the minimum alveolar concentration concept which has proved so fertile. However, the minimum alveolar concentration is a statistical abstraction derived from a group of patients and we need a term to signify the alveolar concentration of agents (when in equilibrium with the brain) at which an individual patient loses motor response to incision. Perhaps 'anaesthetizing alveolar concentration' (AAC) would do.

To approach this subject from a more practical angle, many would consider that 'awareness' could not occur in a patient anaesthetized with an inhalational agent without muscle relaxant and in whom there was no response to surgical incision. This is a reasonable view and there is only one recorded case in which 'awareness' apparently occurred, although all the above criteria had been met.

In this case[15], a 27-year-old man of ASA grade 1 status (where ASA = American Society of Anesthesiology) underwent a revision of hip arthroplasty. Premedication and the anaesthetic technique were conventional and after thiopentone, suxamethonium and tracheal intubation, the patient breathed spontaneously nitrous oxide/oxygen (FIO_2 maintained at 0.3) and halothane, 3.5% at incision descending to 0.6% after 2 hours. At no time in the 3.5-hour operation did the patient move. Blood pressure, pulse rate and blood gases were not abnormal. The next day the patient reported that he had been awake during the operation and was able to support this by repeating surgical conversations which took place at the beginning of the operation and one hour later. No complaint was made of feeling any pain.

Before leaving consideration of the motor response as a marker of position in the anaesthetic continuum, the author would like briefly to return to consideration of the vast numbers of neurones in the central nervous system. In relation to the whole total, the number of motor neurones is quite remarkably small, perhaps two or three million. It is estimated that a typical motor neurone in the spinal cord has perhaps 10 000 synaptic contacts on its surface. These are made up of 2000 on the cell body and 8000 on the dendrites. The motor neurone is therefore the final common pathway from an immense computational network, and whether or not it is stimulated may be a good guide to the presence or absence of consciousness.

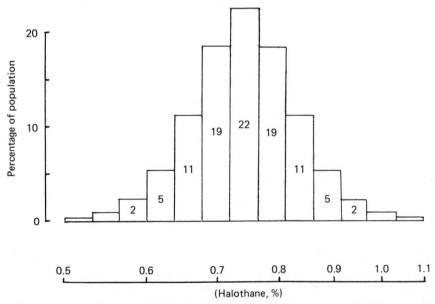

Figure 1.3 The spread of the minimum alveolar concentration in a population of 100 patients. The data are derived from de Jong and Eger[16] and analysed using the logistic equation $y = x^s/(A^s + x^s)$ where A is the minimum alveolar concentration for halothane and s represents the 'steepness' of the S-shaped dose–response curve. For details, *see* Waud[17]

In modern practice, awareness occurs in patients paralysed by muscle relaxants who have not been given sufficient anaesthetic to produce anaesthesia. The reason why it is not possible to be sure that anaesthesia will be produced in an individual patient by a particular concentration of halothane is the spread of sensitivity to the drug in the population. It is possible to measure this spread using the data from which the minimum alveolar concentration has been calculated[16]. It can be seen from *Figure 1.3* that the concentration of halothane needed to anaesthetize the more resistant patient would be dangerous for others. *Figure 1.3* may be said to illustrate the *raison d'être* of anaesthetists.

Finally, how can we ascertain if the patient is anaesthetized or not? One of the principal features of the anaesthetic state is a lack of responsiveness. It seems likely, therefore, that the form of test most likely to succeed is one in which some form of stimulus is applied and the presence, absence or modification of a response is noted, that is an evoked response test. This is exemplified by the minimum alveolar concentration determination, but there are many other possibilities.

One problem is that any measurement of anaesthetic 'depth' seems to be itself affected by surgical stimulus. A solution to this problem would involve some way of quantifying surgical stimuli. It may be that the best that can be done at present is to take a consensus of several different sorts of observation. This would be an extension of existing procedures. The solution to this problem will have a great effect on anaesthetic practice.

Acknowledgements

My thanks are due to Dr M. J. Powers, who drew my attention to the 1771 definition of anaesthesia and to Dr R. S. Cormack who provided *Figure 1.3*.

References

1. WOODBRIDGE, P. D. (1957) Changing concepts concerning depth of anesthesia. *Anesthesiology*, **18**, 536–550
2. *Encyclopaedia Britannica* or *A Dictionary of Arts & Sciences* (1771) by a Society of Gentlemen in Scotland. Printed for A. Bell & Co., MacFarquhar, Edinburgh
3. JONES, J. G., HENEGHAN, C. P. H. and THORNTON, C. (1985) The functional assessment of the normal brain during general anaesthesia. In *Anaesthesia Review 3*, edited by L. Kaufman, pp. 83–98. Edinburgh: Churchill Livingstone
4. TAYLOR, G. R. (1979) *The Natural History of the Mind*. London: Secker & Warburg
5. BLAKEMORE, C. (1977) *Mechanics of the Mind*. Cambridge: Cambridge University Press
6. BENNETT, H. L., DAVIS, H. S. and GIANNINI, J. A. (1985) Non-verbal response to intraoperative conversation. *British Journal of Anaesthesia*, **57**, 174–179
7. LEVINSON, B. W. (1965) States of awareness during general anaesthesia. Preliminary communication. *British Journal of Anaesthesia*, **37**, 544–546
8. WONG, K. C. (1983) Narcotics are not expected to produce unconsciousness and amnesia. *Anesthesia and Analgesia*, **62**, 625–626
9. SAIDMAN, L. J. and EGER, E. I. (1964) Effects of nitrous oxide and of narcotic premedication on the alveolar concentration of halothane required for anesthesia. *Anesthesiology*, **25**, 302–306
10. MUNSON, E. S., SAIDMAN, L. J. and EGER, E. I. (1965) Effect of nitrous oxide and morphine on the minimum anesthetic concentration of fluroxene. *Anesthesiology*, **26**, 134–139
11. MURPHY, M. R. and HUG, C. C. (1982) The enflurane sparing effect of morphine, butorphanol, and nalbuphine. *Anesthesiology*, **57**, 489–492

12. MURPHY, M. R. and HUG, C. C. (1982) The anesthetic potency of fentanyl in terms of its reduction of enflurane MAC. *Anesthesiology*, **57**, 485–488

13. ARTUSIO, J. F. (1955) Ether analgesia during major surgery. *Journal of the American Medical Association*, **157**, 33–36

14. DIXON, N. (1981) *Preconscious Processing*, p. 264. Chichester: John Wiley & Sons

15. SAUCIER, N., WALTS, L. F. and MORELAND, J. R. (1983) Patient awareness during nitrous oxide, oxygen, and halothane anesthesia. *Anesthesia and Analgesia*, **362**, 239–240

16. DE JONG, R. H. and EGER, E. I. II (1975) MAC expanded: AD_{50} and AD_{95} values of common inhalation anesthetics in man. *Anesthesiology*, **42**, 384–389

17. WAUD, D. R. (1972) On biological assays involving quantal responses. *Journal of Pharmacology and Experimental Therapeutics*, **183**, 577–607

Chapter 2

The state of consciousness: some humanistic considerations

E. M. Papper

The emphasis of this book is directed towards identification of those conditions which permit undesirable, and perhaps unexpected, restoration of consciousness during anaesthesia, which is not in the patient's best interest.

This chapter examines some aspects of the state of consciousness and is prompted by thinking about the problems caused by the actions of general anaesthesia, including some of the unpredictable results.

All anaesthetists, and probably all other discerning people, seem to take for granted that there is a clear understanding of what consciousness and awareness are, and why they are to be avoided during the conduct of general anaesthesia. However, further reflection on this problem suggests that such thinking is really based, at least to some degree, upon commonly accepted intuitions in which we tend to agree that we all understand what consciousness and awareness may be. In a sense, efforts at trying to come to grips with this matter are not altogether different from the problems in relation to understanding pain in human beings.

We really find it difficult, if not impossible, to define pain clearly enough, but we tend to relate our understanding of pain to the observations that are provoked by painful experience in people which appears to manifest itself in the form of suffering. Someone else's pain cannot be quantified, but his suffering can be observed. In the same sense, we cannot really share that level of awareness and consciousness in others, but we can share what is probably one of the most basic of human experiences. This human experience is the foundation for all of science and art, all of religion and philosophy and all of thought, no matter how directed or undirected it appears to be at any given moment.

This intuitive notion can perhaps be further extended by stating that to the observer who thinks about these problems, the state of consciousness and awareness is almost the same as, if not entirely coincidental with, a definition of life.

In a very long career of giving clinical anaesthesia to patients, it has also occurred to the author that the removal of consciousness, deliberately and for an alleged, and probably certain, benefit to a patient, does remove for that patient all that the individual knows of life itself. The extension of this perception is the critical responsibility assumed by the anaesthetist for taking into his or her hands all that another individual knows of life and the responsibility for restoring it. Since we seem to have general, although largely intuitive, agreement on what consciousness and awareness may be, we trouble ourselves very little about most of the intellectual and perceptual aspects of this fascinating state which distinguishes human beings from other forms of life, and busy ourselves with the consequences of failure to produce unconsciousness. All these practices and views are entirely understandable and reasonable, but they are really insufficient for the comprehension of a basic problem in biological science.

It may be satisfactory to many to think of consciousness as a religious endowment, which is divinely bestowed and, therefore, for them there is no further need to examine its consequences other than to accept it. It is also possible to think philosophically about consciousness and to accept it as a given postulate and make deductions with pure and logical reason that have validity as long as the basic hypothesis is correct[1].

It seems, however, that these approaches fall short of an adequate understanding of what we are dealing with. Unconsciousness of course can be produced, even with the limited agreement that is intuitional, by injury to the central nervous system, by drugs, by non-pharmacological methods such as hypnosis, and behavioural conditioning. All these modalities seem to demand the question of what is basically affected other than the consensual agreement of intention.

It may be more useful than rewarding to accept the limitations of understanding consciousness and awareness in the way that we seem to have accepted our limitations and understanding of the mechanism of general anaesthesia and, for that matter, the pain experience as well. However, there is the real possibility, with the advances of molecular biology, that an objective approach to a definition of the state of consciousness is a possibility that can be subjected to all of the classical rigours of scientific thought and observed experience, and extend our capabilities beyond those of intuition and the acceptance of given postulates.

It is conceivable, for instance, that the state of consciousness is a matter of the appropriate molecular structure of certain transmitters or perhaps even the sequencing of amino acids somewhere in the central nervous system. If this assumption has any merit, with the advance in modern technology, it may, one day, be susceptible to deliberate examination and development in accordance with human experience that goes beyond that of intuition. Since the anaesthetist is one of the major producers of unconsciousness, it seems no more than reasonable that his disciplines and his methods of work could form the foundation for an objective realistic scientific understanding of consciousness.

This thought is less practical than many in the other chapters but it suggests, at least to this author, that the study of consciousness and awareness could be one of the most fruitful and ambitious areas of research in anaesthesia for the near and long-term future.

We could at least learn whether we have any hope of understanding, in a mechanistic sense, the process of consciousness or whether we must accept the fact that we are left with only an intuition.

Recent studies on memory, which deal in a peripheral way with a state of consciousness, suggest that it is possible to study this particular problem in objective scientific ways and it is to be hoped that it will be one of the areas of interest for future research[2].

References

1. HIMSWORTH, SIR H. (1986) *Scientific Knowledge and Philosophical Thought*. Baltimore: The Johns Hopkins University Press
2. KANDEL, E. (1983) What molecular steps determine the time and course of the memory for short-term sensitization in Aplysia? *Cold Spring Harbor Symposia on Quantitative Biology*, **48**, 811–819

Chapter 3

Detecting consciousness by clinical means

M. D. Vickers

It is clear that one can become confused by the various terms that are being used, not all of which have been defined in a generally accceptable manner. Even the title of the workshop 'Unconsciousness during general anaesthesia' is a tautology if one accepts the everyday meaning of these two concepts.

This chapter is about monitoring unconsciousness. Can one monitor something which is *not* there? What needs to be addressed at a practical level is the ability to detect consciousness or, more strictly, the ability to detect impending consciousness in time to prevent its occurrence.

One difficulty is that we all instinctively know what we mean by the terms 'conscious' and 'unconscious'. However, I am not sure that these can be regarded as opposites or indeed as unitary states. Otherwise one could give no meaning to such concepts as states of altered consciousness.

Likewise, awareness is not strictly a synonym for consciousness. The latter is strictly an experience unique to the individual experiencing it. Awareness can be inferred from behaviour without the experience of consciousness. Thus, attempts to define awareness or consciousness are probably doomed to failure. I propose to cut the gordian knot by first defining unconsciousness, which can be done in a fairly acceptable way as 'No evidence, either at the time or later, of perception, registration or retention of mental images corresponding accurately to real events'. This definition has to be thrown wide to encompass ideomotor behaviour unassociated with any conscious recall, based on suggestions made during supposed unconsciousness.

Given such a definition, I will take as its opposite, not consciousness or awareness, but the semantic purity of 'non-unconsciousness' – a tedious but valuable double negative. The problem which then needs attention is the detection of non-unconsciousness, or its incipient development.

Despite a recent opinion to the contrary[1], I propose to take a very pragmatic line over this and suggest that there are, for all practical purposes, two kinds of non-unconsciousness: the evidence of retention of some aspect of an auditory input; and the recall of actual experiences. This may be too simplistic, but the literature in general does suggest that there are two types of phenomenon either reported or investigated, and that they may *not* be parts of a continuum.

Detecting meaningful auditory inputs

There is an increasing number of reports to support the view that meaningful auditory inputs can and do register in the brain even during apparent surgical anaesthesia[2-5]. If this is true, then this is not a new problem associated with the introduction of muscle relaxants, but must have been at least a potential problem since the discovery of anaesthesia. It has merely been lack of sophistication to detect the phenomenon that makes it seem like a modern problem.

Cheek[6] is the most committed exponent of the view that the brain can and does attend to what is going on under surgical anaesthesia. However, it was Levinson[2], 21 years ago, who first alarmed anaesthetists with the results of an open study involving a piece of play-acting performed for the benefit of patients under ether anaesthesia followed by hypnotic recall of the content of this.

Levinson's paper contains an eight-channel EEG taken in one patient when the disturbing auditory stimulus was applied; this demonstrated a quite abrupt change indicative of attention. No statement was made concerning any clinical signs that could have been picked up by an observant anaesthetist; if there were, Levinson either did not notice them or did not report them.

But an additional problem with this type of non-unconsciousness is that it seems to be a potential state, rather than an actual one. Many investigators have tried a variety of auditory inputs during surgical anaesthesia and sought subsequently for various kinds of evidence to show that they had an effect[2,5-13]. Recall, spontaneous or hypnotically aided, has only rarely been elicited for non-meaningful or neutral material[5,7].

Cheek[6] is quite vehement that only something which is 'perceived' by the anaesthetized patient as relevant to themselves will gain their attention. Bennett, Davis and Giannini[4] chose a message which was personal but not threatening and obtained evidence that the message (to pull the ear-lobe at a post-operative interview) had been received and understood, although it was not remembered. Levinson[2] used an acted 'emergency' which appeared to threaten the life of the patient and which was delivered by the actual anaesthetist as realistically as possible. However, Millar and Watkinson[5] used neutral words versus random noise and showed that these words were significantly better identified by the test group in a subsequently shown 40 word list containing them.

This, and other work, is sufficient for me to accept the hypothesis that auditory inputs *can* be registered by the anaesthetized patient if they are sufficiently significant, and also the hypothesis that, if they are also realistically alarming, the experience may have subtle effects on the unconscious mind.

To come back to the brief for the chapter, however, the total lack of contemporaneous comment by investigators, supplemented by the accumulated 'non-experience' of countless anaesthetists and the millions of patients who have been in this state, makes it almost certain that there is little possibility of detecting clinically a state of 'being able to attend to a meaningful auditory stimulus'. If we believe it does matter, then prevention is the only avenue which is practicable at present. Whether or not it can be reliably detected by some aspect of the EEG, is considered elsewhere in the book.

Recall of actual experiences

Being able spontaneously to recall events occurring during supposed general anaesthesia, whether associated with pain or not, and the ability also to recall the fact of consciousness and the feelings experienced, is a problem of a different order and one which, obviously, ought never to exist unintended. It is possible to give modern inhalational or intravenous agents in concentrations that will ensure the absence of this type of consciousness without any risk of organ toxicity. Why then, do we not use one or other such technique routinely when we use relaxants? In the absence of special reasons or other means for ensuring unconsciousness, not to do so must now be regarded as indefensible. However, even if all anaesthetists at all times gave what they believed to be a reliable level of inhalational agent or an adequate infusion rate of an intravenous agent, the problem would not go away. There is always the chance of accidental underdosing, leaks, machinery malfunction and abnormal resistance to anaesthesia. Any of these occurring in a patient who has received a significant amount of muscle relaxant is nowadays likely to provide a quick short-cut to a claim for damages.

There can be no doubt that, in the absence of special circumstances, the British courts will accept the patient's evidence of recall, if at all confirmable, as a reason for damages. Obtaining damages implies some injury but as far as I know the courts have not delineated what actually constitutes the injury. It is unlikely that the courts are interested in the adverse effects of autonomic activity, even though, short term, this is clearly harmful, with dysrhythmias being an obvious threat to life. As to the more subtle possible long-term ill-effects, the blocking of the catabolic response to surgery has not been shown to have any detectable effect on outcome. So, although being aware during surgery will usually (although not necessarily) be accompanied by autonomic overactivity, from a medicolegal point of view this is not the cause of any 'harm' that comes to the patient. The 'harm' must be regarded as a purely psychic trauma and composed of one or more of three elements: unwillingly experiencing pain, being awake, and being unable to communicate either fact.

Let us consider how the possibility of a clinical indication of consciousness relates to these three aspects.

Pain

Consciously and involuntarily experienced pain must be accompanied by autonomic activity of such an intensity that it would be negligent to ignore it. A major problem, however, is our blasé attitude to signs of less intense sympathetic overactivity. Experience over and over again shows that tachycardia, hypertension, sweating and tear secretion do not necessarily mean that a patient is conscious; in fact, comparatively rarely do they mean this. This inevitably builds the false confidence that they do not have that connotation on *this* occasion. There is, unfortunately, no clear distinction between the intensity of the response to a painful stimulus under light anaesthesia, and the response when conscious, although one would imagine the latter would be worse.

What about the obverse? If we always treated autonomic activity as though it indicated conscious pain, would we abolish the risk of consciousness? It would depend on how we treated it, but, as a generalization, almost certainly not. It is certainly possible to abolish the sensation of pain with sufficient analgesic drug without necessarily abolishing consciousness.

Being awake

There is no obvious inevitable psychic ill-effects of consciousness as such during surgery. Patients are willing to experience some pain and discomfort if their motivation to be awake is sufficiently high. As soon as we come to being awake when both parties had *not* agreed to it, however, then the fact of being awake itself may legitimately be the cause of complaint.

Does unwilling consciousness without any pain stimulate detectable autonomic activity? One must assume that if it generates the requisite emotion, then it will. But, unfortunately, it is all too likely that the anaesthetist will have used one or more other agents which modify emotion, but which do not necessarily make pain-free awareness a pleasant experience. The butyrophenones and some phenothiazines can produce a state of unexpressed inner agitation. Whatever the contemporaneous emotion, however, there is likely to be a retrospective sense of injustice, easily egged on to litigation. It is, in fact, not likely to be a case of 'emotion recollected in tranquillity'.

Inability to communicate

Inability to communicate is not, itself, distressful if the individual realizes that this is an intended and necessary condition of limited duration and receives constant reassurance. It is when a patient believes he or she should actually be unconscious and that the fact that they are not unconscious is not being realized and cannot be communicated, that distress seems likely.

Certainly there have been occasional reports of patients who were aware and not able to communicate, but *not* upset[12]. This possibility will strike most people as surprising. It is commonly thought that being conscious that one ought to be *unconscious* and not able to communicate *would* be upsetting, and indeed the great majority of the reportage supports this view. However, the frequent failure to complain spontaneously suggests that there are grades of being upset and that remembering being conscious is not as upsetting as remembering feeling pain. Remembering that one was frightened probably lies in between.

Recognizing a distress signal

Clearly, a distressing situation need not persist if there is an adequate signal from the patient to the anaesthetist. However, the signal may be weak, or may be ignored, misinterpreted or merely undetected and 'lost' in the background of normal variability.

In the clinical situation there are only two possible signals capable of clinical detection: muscle activity intended to lead to movement and autonomic activity stimulating the sympathetic nervous system.

Muscle movement

Tunstall[14] has sought to rely on muscle movement by excluding some muscles from the effects of relaxants and attempting to communicate with the patient. The technique generally does not seem to have caught on. The bald fact is that, in most reported instances, the anaesthetist has had no indication that the patient was conscious until he learned about it post-operatively.

Logically, there is no reason to suppose that, because no signal was seen or observed, no signal was emitted. It may have been because the patient was too paralysed. In the absence of clinical monitoring of the degree of relaxation, even the most experienced anaesthetist could make such an error. Alternatively, it may have been because relevant movement was impeded, for example, by arm restrainers, or perhaps movement simply was not adequately looked for. Not every anaesthetist manages to keep a close watch on the patient's face at all times. Perhaps patients do not always move the right muscle in a purposive way. Movement may then be interpreted as a reflex, and nothing to do with consciousness.

Again, however, we have the problem of the false positive. All anaesthetists have had experience of patients who moved, often apparently quite purposefully, and yet there has been no subsequent recall. Whenever a lot of false positives (in any field of activity) are experienced, the signal inevitably comes to be ignored. This is a psychological problem, and the only solution would be to treat every peripheral muscle movement as indicating incipient consciousness.

Sympathetic activity

However, one cannot even take this purist line with signs of undue sympathetic activity, at least as far as tachycardia or changes in blood pressure are concerned, since there are several other possible causes. Tear secretion is generally held to indicate too light a level of anaesthesia, but would tears flow for consciousness in the absence of pain? We would certainly speak of tears of frustration. They are a warning sign that the patient is 'too light', but again the obverse is not true. Tears are sometimes secreted without there being any conscious recall. Paradoxically, powerful analgesics have probably been unhelpful since they can abolish the massive autonomic response to pain, but do not necessarily suppress the lesser response to unwilling consciousness, which is harder to detect when pain is not present.

Detection or warning?

What has been considered above is the chance of detecting consciousness by clinical means. However, even if we could develop an absolutely reliable method, it would be a useless exercise until we develop a drug to produce retrograde amnesia. It would be a classic case of shutting the stable door after the horse had bolted; until we have a reliable retrograde amnesic all we can do by such an approach is to limit the possibility of any *further* consciousness. What is needed is not an indicator of consciousness, but an indicator that consciousness is about to be gained, in time to prevent its onset. This is a limitation which may hobble efforts with any monitoring system, however sophisticated. Linked to this is the problem of the effect of changes in surgical stimulation on the level of consciousness.

Potential benefits?

While it seems impossible that recall of unintended consciousness can have any benefits, the possibility of the registration of meaningful auditory inputs might be turned to advantage[15]. Indeed, there is already a report[16] (unfortunately of an inadequately controlled trial) concluding that suitable suggestions given during general anaesthesia reduced the need for post-operative analgesics. This is work which would bear repeating in a properly controlled fashion.

Conclusions

There is a considerable body of reportage pointing to the ability of the brain to monitor what it hears down to quite respectable levels of general anaesthesia. Provided, however, that the material is neutral or positively beneficial there is no evidence that this does any harm.

With regard to recalled awareness, all that can be said is that *if* we never completely paralyse the patient, and if we carefully observe all aspects of his or her behaviour critically, and if on every occasion we use a technique which has been shown to minimize the risk of consciousness, and if we monitor every patient by expired air analysis or EEG analysis as appropriate, we ought not to discover any patient that has recall. Unfortunately we do not.

References

1. JONES, J. G. and KONIECZO, K. (1986) Hearing and memory in anaesthetised patients. *British Medical Journal*, **292**, 1291–1293
2. LEVINSON, B. W. (1965) States of awareness during general anaesthesia. Preliminary communication. *British Journal of Anaesthesia*, **37**, 544–546
3. CHEEK, D. B. (1964) Further evidence of persistence of hearing under chemo-anesthesia: detailed case report. *American Journal of Clinical Hypnosis*, **7**, 55–59
4. BENNETT, H. L., DAVIS, H. S. and GIANNINI, J. A. (1985) Non-verbal response to intraoperative conversation. *British Journal of Anaesthesia*, **57**, 174–179
5. MILLAR, K. and WATKINSON, N. (1983) Recognition of words presented during general anaesthesia. *Ergonomics*, **26**, 585–594
6. CHEEK, D. B. (1979) Awareness of meaningful sounds under general anaesthesia: considerations and a review of the literature 1959–1979. Paper presented at the 1979 Annual Scientific meeting of the American Society of Clinical Hypnosis. Reprints available from Symposia Specialists, 1470 N. E. 129th Street, Miami, Florida, 33161, *Theoretical and Clinical Aspects of Hypnosis*
7. McINTYRE, J. W. R. (1966) Awareness during general anaesthesia: preliminary observations. *Canadian Anaesthetists' Society Journal*, **13**, 495–499
8. BRICE, D. D., HETHERINGTON, R. R. and UTTING, J. E. (1970) A simple study of awareness and dreaming during anaesthesia. *British Journal of Anaesthesia*, **42**, 535–541
9. TERRELL, R. K., SWEET, W. O., GLADFELTER, J. H. and STEPHEN, C. R. (1969) Study of recall during anesthesia. *Anesthesia and Analgesia*, **48**, 86–90
10. ABRAMSON, M., GREENFIELD, I. and HERON, W. T. (1966) Response to or perception of auditory stimuli under deep surgical anesthesia. *American Journal of Obstetrics and Gynecology*, **96**, 584–587
11. CRAWFORD, J. S., LEWIS, M. AND DAVIES, P. (1985) Maternal and neonatal responses related to the volatile agent used to maintain anaesthesia at Caesarean section. *British Journal of Anaesthesia*, **57**, 482–487
12. SIA, R. L. (1969) Consciousness during general anaesthesia. *Anesthesia and Analgesia*, **48**, 363–366
13. HUTCHINSON, R. (1961) Awareness during surgery. A study of its incidence. *British Journal of Anaesthesia*, **33**, 463–469
14. TUNSTALL, M. E. (1977) Detecting wakefulness during general anaesthesia for caesarean section. *British Medical Journal*, **1**, 1321
15. PEARSON, R. E. (1961) Response to suggestions given under general anesthesia. *American Journal of Clinical Hypnosis*, **4**, 106–114
16. WOLFE, L. S. and MILLET, J. B. (1960) Control of post-operative pain by suggestion under general anesthesia. *American Journal of Clinical Hypnosis*, **3**, 109–114

Chapter 4

Clinical signs and autonomic responses

John M. Evans

'The signs of anaesthesia have for a long time and with good reason been regarded as fundamental knowledge for anaesthetists. Without a knowledge of these "signs" it would be a foolhardy anaesthetist indeed who would take his patient on a journey from life towards death called anaesthesia. No motorist would set out without a map of his route and without feeling able to recognise a few important landmarks on the way to his destination; yet the responsibility of the motorist is far less onerous than that of the anaesthetist.'

The above is an eloquent description of the significance of the clinical signs of anaesthesia[1]. They serve not only to protect the patient from overdosage of anaesthetic, which was understandably a great concern in the early days of anaesthesia, but equally to protect the patient from the risk of underdosage and the possibility that he may have recall of events during anaesthesia, a possibility which increasingly preoccupies contemporary anaesthetists.

There is a widespread belief that clinical signs have no part to play in assessing the adequacy or depth of modern anaesthesia[2]. Such a view is not consistent with the fact that clinical signs have been virtually the only means by which anaesthetists have successfully controlled many millions of anaesthetics over the years. They are by no means foolproof[3, 4], and the fact that approximately 1% of patients are aware during anaesthesia gives some indication of their (or the anaesthetist's) limitations[5]. Nevertheless, they can be at least as effective as any other single means for providing a guide to the depth of anaesthesia.

The following is part of an account provided by a patient who was aware during a caesarean section[6].

'It was bad from the onset, and it increased in severity. In character it was exceedingly unpleasant. The nearest comparison would be the pain of a tooth drilled without local anaesthetic – when the drill hits a nerve. *Multiply* this pain so that the area involved would equal a thumb-print, then pour a steady stream of molten lead into it. If you imagine the effect of a too-hot pan moved from the cooker onto a plastic surface, then that is what that pain is doing to my non-existent body. Searing, melting, pressing me into the table, with a nasty reminder of a dentist's drill. It never stopped, or wavered in intensity, except in becoming increasingly more unbearable.'

It may well be difficult to detect a limited degree of awareness by observing changes in clinical signs but, providing a patient is not pharmacologically or physiologically compromised, it is hard to believe that a patient experiencing awareness as described above would not generate some manifestation of their distress by significant changes in their clinical signs; equally it is probable that careful observation of clinical signs would offer the patient some protection from this experience.

Historical considerations

Early anaesthetists clearly paid great attention to details of clinical signs[7]. Their concern was to ensure that the patient did not move, was appropriately relaxed and, probably of greatest importance, that the patient was not approaching impending death[8]. The signs generally observed included: pulse quality, colour, muscle tone, respiration, and eye signs.

In 1934, Guedel described his classification of clinical signs for ether anaesthesia which remained a foundation for inhalational anaesthetics[9]. Guedel's classification relied almost completely upon skeletal muscle activity. Despite this, it perfectly fulfilled the requirements for ether anaesthesia as then employed.

The introduction of muscle relaxants

In 1945, a *Lancet* editorial gave an indication of the problem that the use of muscle relaxation was to provide[10]:

'When using curare, the anaesthetist soons learns that those reflexes he calls "the signs of anaesthesia" can no longer be elicited, however little general anaesthetic has been given. They form no guide as to whether his patient is feeling pain or is unconscious. Care must be taken to deaden sensation and ensure unconsciousness, or the worst imaginings of the novelist may come true, for the patient can give no sign if the general anaesthetic is ineffective.'[1]

Initially, muscle relaxants were used to supplement inhalational anaesthesia, with spontaneous ventilation as a means of producing muscle relaxation; the practice of producing complete muscle relaxation and subsequent reversal developed over the next decade.

Since muscle relaxation could now be obtained without recourse to deep inhalational anaesthesia, it was not long before nitrous oxide alone or supplemented by intravenous pethidine was employed to produce anaesthesia. The difficulty is in determining the degree of anaesthesia, and the possibility of patient awareness soon followed[11,12].

With the loss of the classic clinical signs of inhalational anaesthesia, it is surprising that there was little obvious effort directed towards establishing some means for assessing the adequacy of anaesthesia in a paralysed patient. A contemporary review of the signs of anaesthesia by Mushin in 1959 was still dominated by reference to Guedel's concepts and only the briefest reference to the use of autonomic signs was made[1].

In the early days of anaesthesia, the anaesthetist was in close contact with the patient; he could see and hear breathing, he would feel the peripheral pulse, the colour and perfusion of the skin was noted and the eyes carefully observed. The modern anaesthetist is becoming increasingly distanced from the patient; access to the patient's face may be impossible, the eyes are covered by protective tape and physical contact is minimal. Clinical signs *are* important and should not be obscured or ignored, every reasonable effort should be exerted to ensure that potentially useful clinical signs are accessible.

General considerations

Effects of surgery

Surgery is trauma and the physiological response to surgery is essentially the same as to any other trauma. The immediate response of a patient experiencing surgery without anaesthesia would include the following: movement (limb retraction, facial grimacing), myotonia, hyperventilation, hypertension, tachycardia, sweating, lacrimation, and mydriasis.

The responses are partly voluntary, mostly executed by skeletal muscles, and partly involuntary, mostly executed by autonomic mechanisms as a predominantly sympathetic stress response. A conscious perception and reaction to the circumstances will augment these responses; suppression of consciousness may only partly reduce the response.

Effects of anaesthesia

The response of a patient to a typical anaesthetic in the absence of surgery would include: cessation of voluntary movement, muscle relaxation, hypoventilation, hypotension, heart rate (variable response), suppression of sweating, suppression of lacrimation and miosis. This response is somewhat idealized but serves to indicate that the pharmacodynamic effects of many anaesthetics tend to be directly opposite to those produced by surgical stimulus.

For the purpose of this consideration, and as a generalization, the effects of anaesthetic agents can be categorized:

- They act on the central nervous system to produce unconsciousness, their primary therapeutic function.
- They have a secondary analgesic action which attenuates the stress response to surgery.
- They may have specific effects upon individual physiological systems.

The primary action is clearly mandatory, the secondary action is usually desirable and the third effect is generally regarded as an undesirable side-effect.

Properties of anaesthetic agents

Not all drugs used in contemporary anaesthesia have a similar pattern of activity. It is important that this is fully appreciated, since an anaesthetist familiar with the subtleties of one particular agent may encounter very great difficulty in the interpretation of clinical signs when a new and unfamiliar drug with a different pattern of activity is used. Some generalizations along the following lines can be made to categorize agents.

Good anaesthetics, poor analgesics

An anaesthetic may have a powerful primary narcotic effect (narcosis, as distinct from analgesia) and have little accompanying secondary analgesic activity. The intravenous agents thiopentone and etomidate are examples; although unconsciousness is easily achieved with these agents, surgery generates marked reflex activity which can only be successfully suppressed by large doses of the drug. If the anaesthetist achieves significant suppression of the response to surgery with these agents, it is more than likely that a significant excess of drug above that required to produce unconsciousness is given and thus the risks of the patient being aware would be relatively small. However, should the patient become conscious then it is likely that, in the absence of analgesia, the patient's recall of events would include pain and this would render the experience particularly unpleasant.

Poor anaesthetics, good analgesics

Drugs with marked analgesic properties have been used as sole anaesthetic agents. The analgesic agents, in particular morphine and fentanyl, have been used for this purpose, most especially for open heart surgery[13]. Despite the use of very high doses of these drugs, patients have remained aware of events, but it is interesting to note that such accounts of awareness do not generally make reference to pain, stress or discomfort and are composed predominantly of auditory recall[14, 15]. Thus the use of powerful analgesics as anaesthetics agents is likely to be associated with a greater incidence of awareness but, should the patient be aware, it is likely that pain would not be a feature of the experience.

Agents with marked side-effects

Drugs, which have marked side-effects and which produce substantial changes in clinical signs, can prove very difficult to control. For example, an agent which produces a rise in blood pressure and pulse rate (such as ketamine, cyclopropane, fluroxene) may lead the anaesthetist unfamiliar with the agent to regard this as evidence of light anaesthesia and inappropriately to increase the supply of drug to the patient. Conversely, an agent with a marked depressant effect upon the cardiovascular system may lead the anaesthetist into inappropriate reduction in the drug supply with the consequent risk of awareness.

Characteristics of clinical signs

Clinical signs as physiological signals are far from ideal. The control engineers desire for an accurately measured signal is possible for blood pressure and heart rate, but for most other signs accurate measurement is not easy. In brief, clinical signs have the following characteristics:

- Anaesthesia and surgery produce changes which are often, but not always, opposite.
- They are usually qualitative.
- If quantitative, there is often much patient-to-patient variation in absolute values.
- The dose–response, or stimulus–response, curve is variable.
- The response may exhibit fatigue with time.
- The response may exhibit hysteresis.
- Individual clinical responses are often interactive with others (blood pressure and heart rate).
- They are susceptible to interference by many autonomically active drugs.

Interaction of surgery and anaesthesia

It is clear that the interaction of anaesthesia and surgery may well produce a very complex pattern of clinical signs (*Figure 4.1*). Despite this, anaesthetists are clearly successful in using clinical signs to control the majority of anaesthetic procedures. There is, however, very little clinical evidence of the primary narcotic effect of anaesthetics in paralysed patients, and it is probable that the anaesthetist relies upon the secondary effect of the agent to provide clues as to the adequacy of anaesthesia. The tertiary effects of the anaesthetics add 'noise' to this information and render clinical signs more difficult to interpret; anaesthetics with marked side-effects in practice prove more difficult to control.

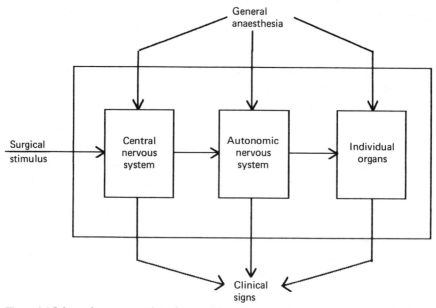

Figure 4.1 Schematic representation of some of the interactions between general anaesthesia, surgical stimulus and clinical signs

Clinical signs and control of anaesthesia

The anaesthetist is a controller; his primary responsibilities are controlling the appropriate supply of anaesthetic agent to the patient together with preserving vital functions.

A naive anaesthetist could be given a set of instructions, or programme, to perform an anaesthetic according to a prescription or recipe[16]. Such a control process, as might be found in an automatic washing machine, is referred to as a feed-forward control system (*Figure 4.2*). It is clear that such a control strategy has limitations. In practice, the anaesthetist commences control of the anaesthetic supply according to a pre-planned regimen, but notes the patient's responses to anaesthesia and surgery and modifies the supply appropriately (*Figure 4.3*). The changes in clinical signs constitute feedback which the anaesthetist uses to modify

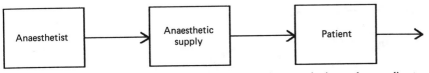

Figure 4.2 Feed-forward control; the anaesthetist controls the anaesthetic supply according to a pre-existing plan

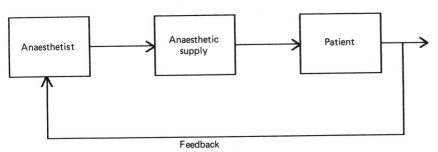

Figure 4.3 Feed-back control; the anaesthetist uses information generated by the patient (clinical signs) to modify his planned control of the anaesthetic supply

his regimens; this constitutes a form of adaptive control. The observation and interpretation of changes in clinical signs is essential if the anaesthetic supply is to be adjusted optimally.

Current clinical practice

Despite the manifest problems inherent in using clinical signs to assess the depth of anaesthesia, there can be no doubt that they are of value. The following points are significant: the anaesthetist collects and successfully uses information contained in the clinical signs; little reliance is placed on any single clinical sign observed in isolation; in the aggregate, the information is of value.

The clinician has skills in the detection and processing of subtle clinical information; if these skills and functions could be identified and replicated in a computer monitoring system, it would be called an expert system.

There are two simple means for information processing: signal summation and signal evaluation.

Signal summation

The individual clinical signs are quantified and summated (*Figure 4.4*). Processing the information in this way has certain consequences: an increase in the value of one sign alone will add only that amount to the sum total; an increase in the value of one sign may be fully offset by a decrease in the value of another making no change to the sum total; a simultaneous increase in all signs will create accordingly larger change in the sum.

In effect, the summation of signals tends to ignore small random changes in individual signs but more clearly identifies mass trends (*see Figure 4.4*).

Signal evaluation and selection

The clinical signs can be observed for a period of time in relation to the conduct of the anaesthetic and surgery until one or more signs are identified which appear to

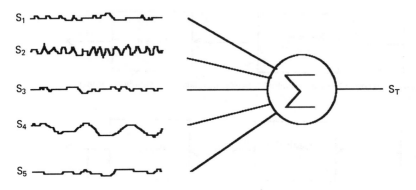

$$S_T = \Sigma (S_1 + S_2 + S_3 + S_4 + S_5)$$

Figure 4.4 Summation of clinical signs. Signs (S_{1-5}) are summated to produce a single index (S_T)

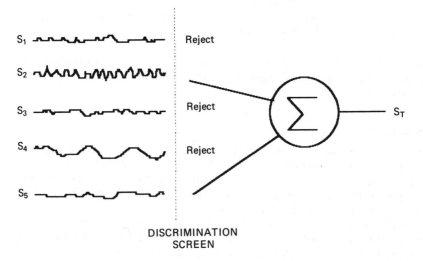

$$S_T = \Sigma (S_2 + S_5)$$

Figure 4.5 Discrimination and summation of clinical signs. The anaesthetist identifies what he believes to be useful signs (e.g. S_2 and S_5), summates them and rejects the other signs

be behaving in the manner expected of an indicator of the adequacy of anaesthesia. This sign (or summated signs if there are more than one) is then used as the preferred indicator thereafter (*Figure 4.5*).

It is likely that anaesthetists use at least both of these approaches together with other processing tricks to enable the interpretation of signs. The second method necessitates that the clinical information be observed for a time, and be subject to an evaluation in which its potential contribution is assessed in relation to the progress of the anaesthetic and surgical procedure. This is a relatively complex task as compared to the former method in which all of the available information is summated.

An approach to evaluating clinical signs using an integrated scoring system for use in paralysed, ventilated patients was described[17], based on the signal summation approach.

An integrated clinical scoring system

Four indices were selected for integration (PRST score): systolic blood pressure (P), heart rate (R), sweating (S), and tear formation (T).

Movement was ignored since this is dependent upon the degree of muscle paralysis and pupil signs were likewise ignored because of their susceptibility to the effect of analgesics. Of the four indices used, two (pressure, rate) are quantitative and objective, while sweating and tears are qualitative and subjectively assessed. Each of the four indices is assigned a score value of 0, 1 or 2 (*see Table 4.1*), so that a sum of the scores has values in the range 0–8. In practice, the mid-point of the range is seldom exceeded and this reflects the redundancy within the scoring system.

Table 4.1 The PRST scale

Index	Condition	Score
Systolic pressure (mmHg)	< Control +15	0
	< Control +30	1
	> Control +30	2
Heart rate (beats/min)	< Control +15	0
	< Control +30	1
	> Control +30	2
Sweating	Nil	0
	Skin moist to touch	1
	Visible beads of sweat	2
Tears	No excess of tears in open eye	0
	Excess of tears in open eye	1
	Tear overflow from closed eye	2

It is assumed that the changes in clinical indices derive from the interaction of anaesthesia and surgery, and that the anaesthetic itself does not have a clinically significant effect upon the individual indices within the score system. If anaesthesia has significant side-effects upon these indices, for example, as produced by ketamine, then the use of this scoring system would be inappropriate.

The threshold values chosen for scoring blood pressure and heart rate are value judgements which are considered to be similar to the corresponding changes described for sweating and tears. It is probable that further refinements of the processing of the P and R components of the score is possible.

The PRST score may be employed in one of two ways: first, it may be employed to control an intermittent incremental supply of drug to a patient. The anaesthetist selects a PRST score threshold which, when equalled or exceeded, indicates the need for an additional increment of drug, for example, an increment of intravenous fentanyl (*Figure 4.6*). This method tends to give rise to a 'saw-tooth' pattern of clinical signs.

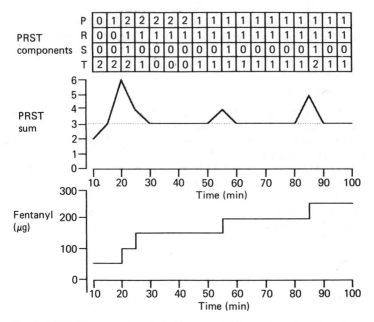

PRST components																				
P	0	1	2	2	2	2	2	1	1	1	1	1	1	1	1	1	1	1		
R	0	0	1	1	1	1	1	1	1	1	1	1	1	1	1	1	1	1		
S	0	0	1	0	0	0	0	0	0	0	1	0	0	0	0	0	0	1	0	0
T	2	2	2	1	0	0	0	0	1	1	1	1	1	1	1	1	2	1	1	

Figure 4.6 PRST score and control of incremental fentanyl supply. When the sum PRST score exceeds the threshold PRST score of 3, an increment of fentanyl is injected. The components of the PRST are shown at the top, the sum PRST in the middle and the cumulative dosage of fentanyl at the bottom

A second strategy employs the PRST score as a means for adjusting a continuous supply of drug to the patient. This essentially amounts to a closed-loop control system (*Figure 4.7*). The anaesthetist selects a set-point or desired PRST score value ($PRST_{set}$) at which the patient is to be maintained. The PRST score is then recorded at intervals (approximately every 5 minutes). If the current recorded PRST ($PRST_{now}$) is greater than the set point, then that is an indication to increase the supply of drug to the patient; if the $PRST_{now}$ is less than $PRST_{set}$, then the

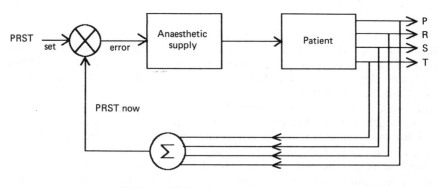

Error = ($PRST_{set}$ − $PRST_{now}$)

Figure 4.7 PRST score and closed-loop control. The summed PRST score ($PRST_{now}$) is compared to the desired score value ($PRST_{set}$). The value of the error signal is used to adjust the anaesthetic supply to the patient to maintain the PRST score at the set value

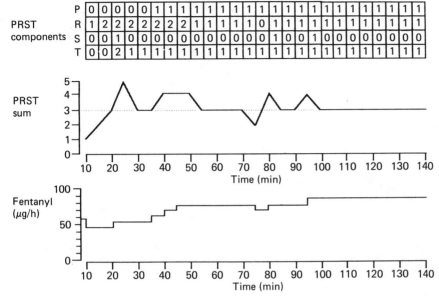

Figure 4.8 PRST score and closed-loop control. The PRST components are shown at the top, the sum PRST in the centre and the infusion rate of fentanyl at the bottom. The PRST$_{set}$ was 3 and the infusion was started at 58 µg/h and adjusted to maintain the measured PRST at the set point

supply of drug to the patient is reduced. The difference between PRST$_{now}$ and PRST$_{set}$ is referred to as the error signal and this can be used to calculate appropriate changes to the drug supply.

Figure 4.8 shows the changing infusion rates of fentanyl for a patient in whom the infusion of fentanyl as a supplement to nitrous oxide was controlled by the PRST score applying the following simple control equation:

$$NR = OR(1 - KE/t)$$

where NR = new infusion rate, OR = old infusion rate, K = a constant (e.g. 0.5), t = time in minutes since last revision, $E = (PRST_{set} - PRST_{now})$.

Anaesthesia was induced with thiopentone, fentanyl (1 µg/kg) with pancuronium. The lungs were ventilated with nitrous oxide 70% and an infusion of fentanyl commenced at 10 minutes. The infusion of fentanyl was set initially to 1 µg/kg per hour but was adjusted at 5-minute intervals according to the control equation above (*Figure 4.9*). After 60 minutes of anaesthesia, one patient had received 24 µg while another had received 80 µg, a range ratio of over 3:1. All patients awoke rapidly; the mean time to obeying commands from cessation of anaesthesia, and an injection of atropine and neostigmine, was 3.9 minutes.

Limitations of clinical signs

The textbook physiological responses constituting the clinical signs have numerous limitations. The response of a single physiological variable in one patient may fall within a very wide range for the population. Clinical signs may further be substantially modified by drug therapy, disease and other factors.

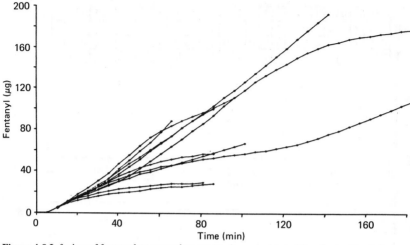

Figure 4.9 Infusion of fentanyl as a supplement to nitrous oxide in 10 patients. The infusion rate was recalculated every 5 minutes according to the equation in the text; the vertical scale shows the cumulative fentanyl dose

Drug therapy

Many interactions are possible. Some examples of potential interactions are listed:

- Anticholinergics – tachycardia, reduced sweating and lacrimation.
- Antihypertensives – reduced pressor responses, possible tachycardia.
- Adrenergic blockers – reduced cardiovascular responses to surgical stimulation, bradycardia, hypotension.
- Adrenergic agonist – exaggerated cardiovascular responses, e.g. bronchodilators, uterine relaxants.
- Psychotropic drugs – many diverse and complex responses are possible with both increase or decrease of autonomic responses, for example lithium, tricyclic antidepressants, monoamine-oxidase inhibitors.
- Benzodiazepines – myotonia.
- Analgesics – potential interaction of agonist and mixed agonist–antagonist analgesics.
- Ophthalmic drugs, which cause miosis (e.g. pilocarpine) or mydriasis (e.g. phenylephrine).
- Drug addiction – drug interaction or withdrawal may generate bizarre signs.

Diseases

The disturbance of normal physiological responses by disease can substantially modify clinical signs:

- Autonomic neuropathy – common in diabetics, may modify many clinical responses.
- Ophthalmic disease – corneal opacities can obscure pupil while neurological lesions may interfere with the normal reflexes (Argyll Robertson pupil).
- Restrictive cardiovascular disease – restrictive valve disease, conduction block or pacemakers can modify cardiovascular signs.

- Respiratory disease can limit the respiratory responses in a non-paralysed patient.
- Central neurological disease, paraplegia, or tetraplegia obviously limit skeletal muscle responses, but spinal hyper-reflexia may be present.
- Hypothermia mimics, if not causes, deepening anaesthesia.
- Endocrine, hypothyroidism and suppression of the pituitary–adrenal function limits or prevents a stress response.

Differential diagnosis of clinical signs

The clinical signs of lightening anaesthesia may also be produced by other conditions. If the signs develop unexpectedly, then the following differential diagnosis should be considered while the adequacy of the anaesthetic supply is verified: hypercarbia, hypoxia, hyperpyrexia, thyrotoxicosis, injection of wrong drug (adrenaline), porphyria, phaeochromocytoma, or carcinoid tumour.

If unexpected evidence of deepening anaesthesia should develop then the anaesthetic supply should be checked and consideration should be given to some of the possible differential diagnoses: hypotension, hypoxia, surgically induced reflex – bradycardia, hypovolaemia, accidental injection of the wrong drug or hypothermia.

Clearly numerous other causes of sudden cardiorespiratory depression or failure are possible.

Specific clinical signs and responses

Respiratory signs

The minute volumes give some indication of the adequacy of anaesthesia in the non-paralysed patient. The detailed changes in the pattern of respiratory muscle activity are fully documented in the descriptions of Guedel and others[18]. Hiccoughs may occur as a feature of light anaesthesia, but considerable deepening of the anaesthesia may subsequently be necessary in order to suppress the response. During anaesthesia, the regularity of the respiratory cycle is increased; minor variations in respiratory rhythmicity are associated with arousal reactions in the EEG[19]. Bronchospasm may develop in the intubated patient and, as with hiccoughs, may only be suppressed by considerable deepening of the anaesthetic.

Cardiovascular signs

The changes in blood pressure and heart rate are well recognized[20]. Changes in cardiac output may also parallel these responses and may be recognized by changes in the peripheral perfusion or capillary oozing at the wound. Auscultation of the heart may reveal a corresponding increase or decrease in the cardiac sounds. The beat-to-beat variation in heart rate decreases during anaesthesia, but this index can become confusing as a result of dysrhythmias resulting from minor conduction changes induced by the anaesthetic agents[21,22]. Changes in the peripheral perfusion, as detected by a pulse plethysmograph, also give some indication of changing peripheral adrenergic activity[23].

Ophthalmic signs

Pupil signs are potentially very useful, but are frequently obscured by the use of narcotic analgesics and their central action on the Edinger–Westphal nucleus. Adequate anaesthesia is usually associated with a moderately small pupil which increases as either anaesthesia deepens or lightens[24]. Pupil eccentricity may develop with overdosage of volatile agents. The pupillary response to light is a characteristic of inadequate anaesthesia and is generally suppressed by most volatile agents at around 2.0 MAC (MAC = minimum alveolar concentration)[25].

Eyelid retraction may develop from excess sympathetic stimulation of the smooth muscle component of the levator palpebrae muscle of the upper eyelid.

Lacrimation is a sign of light anaesthesia and probably arises partly as a response to pain and partly as a response to airway irritation produced either by irritant vapours or by a tracheal tube. It is commonly seen during intubation under light anaesthesia.

Ocular microtremor can be recorded from the globe of the eye as an oscillation of the extraocular muscles arising from the gaze control mechanism in the brainstem[26]. This provides some indication of brainstem activity but, unfortunately, these muscles are exquisitely sensitive to the effect of skeletal muscle relaxants.

The electroretinogram (ERG) is a recently described measurement which is sensitive to anaesthesia and hypoxia[27].

Numerous subtle eye and associated facial signs have been described as an adjunct to Guedel's signs for ether anaesthesia[28].

Skin signs

Skin colour, perfusion and temperature reflect cardiovascular function and oxygenation. The exocrine activity of the sweat glands is controlled by sympathetic pathways although the postganglionic fibres are cholinergic. Increased sweating is a feature of light anaesthesia, but is infrequently seen with most volatile agents and more likely to be encountered during nitrous oxide–narcotic anaesthesia; the narcotic agents have a variable diaphoretic effect which may augment the response. Sweating is usually observed on either the palms or face, but is not confined to these areas. The effects of environmental humidity and temperature are obviously relevant.

Changes in skin impedance may arise before clinically discernible sweating has developed and this gives rise to the changing electrical properties of the skin observed in the pyschogalvanic skin response (PSG)[29].

Sweat production has been estimated by means of an evaporimeter. This is a quantitative response which may prove to be useful in future studies of the stress response[30].

Alimentary tract signs

During light inhalational anaesthesia, swallowing and vomiting can occur; in the intubated patient swallowing or attempted mastication may be seen. In animals, studies of the swallowing reflex indicate a clear suppression with anaesthetic depth[31]. Oesophageal motility is also related to anaesthetic dosage and is referred to elsewhere (Chapter 13). Gastrointestinal activity can be monitored by auscultation of the bowel sounds and is progressively suppressed during deepening anaesthesia[32]. Salivary and other secretions are progressively suppressed by deepening anaesthesia.

Skeletal muscle responses

Cessation of skeletal muscle response in response to surgery is generally taken as an indicator of satisfactory anaesthesia. This is the sign on which measurements of the minimum alveolar concentration depend, and it is a very important yardstick in clinical measurement. The minimum alveolar concentration cannot be measured if the patient is paralysed. The isolated forearm technique described by Tunstall[33] can be used to circumvent this disadvantage. The forearm circulation is isolated by means of a tourniquet applied before skeletal muscle relaxants have been administered and this allows observation of the muscle activity of the arm to be made in the otherwise fully paralysed patient. It has been shown by this means that considerable skeletal muscle activity may be present during skeletal general anaesthesia judged adequate by other means. It is in fact possible to reduce the supply of anaesthetic to the patient to the extent that, not only is involuntary reflex activity present, but voluntary activity can be demonstrated and patients can be instructed to move their hand in response to verbal commands. This is certainly a potentially valuable technique, the application of which is still being explored[34].

Most anaesthetic agents reduce muscle tone. Transient increases may be observed with certain induction agents (e.g. methohexitone), while ketamine produces a sustained increase in tone; in large doses fentanyl may also cause an increase in tone.

The electrical activity of the frontalis muscle has been used as an indicator of anaesthesia depth in the partly paralysed patient (*see* Chapters 10 and 11).

Clinical records

As a matter of routine, the anaesthetist frequently observes many clinical signs – typically, blood pressure, pulse rate, sweating, lacrimation, pupil size and movement. It is usual to record blood pressure and pulse rate, but it is not common practice to record other clinical signs. It could be argued that there is a good case for doing so (*Figure 4.10*). First, in order that the clinical practice of regularly checking the patient is reinforced; secondly, to prompt the anaesthetist into making an assessment of the significance of his observations; and, finally, to demonstrate that the anaesthetist has conducted the care of the patient with full diligence. This should go some way towards providing a defence in the event that negligence is implied.

		5	10	15	20	25	30	35	40	45	50	55	60
Sweat	0, 1, 2	0	0	0	0	0	1	0	0	0	0	0	0
Tears	0, 1, 2	0	0	0	0	1	1	0	0	0	0	0	1
Pupils	mm	2	2	2	2	3	3	2	2	2	2	2	3
Movement	−/+	−	−	−	−	−	+	−	−	−	−	−	−

Figure 4.10 Possible recording scheme for clinical signs as a supplement to conventional anaesthetic records. Sweat and tears are assigned score values according to the changes described in *Table 4.1*. Movement is indicated when it occurs

References

1. MUSHIN, W. W. (1959) Signs of anaesthesia. In *General Anaesthesia*, edited by F. T. Evans and T. C. Gray, pp. 375–387. London: Butterworths
2. WILSON, M. E. (1981) Detection of wakefulness during general anaesthesia. *British Journal of Anaesthesia*, **53**, 1234
3. BAHL, C. P. and WADAS, S. (1968) Consciousness during apparent surgical anaesthesia. A case report. *British Journal of Anaesthesia*, **40**, 289–291
4. SAUCIER, N., WALTS, L. F. and MORELAND, J. R. (1983) Patient awareness during nitrous oxide, oxygen, and halothane anesthesia. *Anesthesia and Analgesia*, **62**, 239–240
5. BRECKENRIDGE, J. L. and AITKENHEAD, A. R. (1983) Awareness during anaesthesia: a review. *Annals of the Royal College of Surgeons of England*, **65**, 93–96
6. EDITORIAL (1979) On being aware. *British Journal of Anaesthesia*, **51**, 711–712
7. SNOW, J. (1847) *On the Inhalation of the Vapour of Ether*. London: Churchill
8. SANSON, A. E. (1885) *Chloroform*. London: Churchill
9. GUEDEL, A. E. (1937) *Inhalational Anesthesia – A Fundamental Guide*. New York: Macmillan
10. EDITORIAL (1945) Curare in anaesthesia. *Lancet*, **ii**, 81–82
11. WINTERBOTTOM, E. H. (1950) Insufficient anaesthesia. *British Medical Journal*, **1**, 247–248
12. SIKER, E. S. (1956) Analgesic supplements to nitrous oxide anesthesia. *British Medical Journal*, **2**, 1326–1331
13. MOLDENHAUER, C. C. and HUG, C. C. (1984) Use of narcotic analgesics as anaesthetics. *Clinics in Anesthesiology*, **2**, 107–343
14. HILGENBERG, J. C. (1981) Intraoperative awareness during high-dose fentanyl–oxygen anesthesia. *Anesthesiology*, **54**, 341–343
15. WONG, K. G. (1983) Narcotics are not expected to produce unconsciousness and amnesia. *Anesthesia and Analgesia*, **62**, 625–626
16. CHILCOAT, R. T. (1980) A review of the control of depth of anaesthesia. *Transactions of the Institute of Measurement and Control*, **2**, 38–45
17. EVANS, J. M., FRASER, A., WISE, C. C. and DAVIES, W. L. (1983) Computer controlled anesthesia. In: *Computing in Anaesthesia and Intensive Care*, edited by O. Prakash, pp. 279–291. Boston: Martinus Nijhoff
18. ARTUSIO, J. F., CORSENN, G., DORNETTE, W. H. L. and REEVES, J. G. (1972) Monitoring depth of anesthesia. In *Legal Aspects of Anaesthesia*, pp. 212–222. Philadelphia: F. A. Davis Company
19. BIMAR, J. and BELLVILLE, J. W. (1977) Arousal reactions during anesthesia in man. *Anesthesiology*, **47**, 449–454
20. KISSIN, I. and GREEN, D. (1984) Effect of halothane on cardiac acceleration response to somatic nerve stimulation in dogs. *Anesthesiology*, **54**, 708–711
21. SAVEGE, T. M., DUBOIS, M., FRANK, M. and HOLLY, J. M. P. (1978) Preliminary investigation into a new method of assessing the quality of anaesthesia: the cardiovascular response to a measured noxious stimulus. *British Journal of Anaesthesia*, **50**, 481–488
22. CARTER, R. T. and ASBURY, A. J. (1983) Heart rate variability and anaesthesia. *British Journal of Anaesthesia*, **55**, 916P
23. JOHNSTONE, M. (1974) Digital vasodilatation: a sign of anaesthesia. *British Journal of Anaesthesia*, **46**, 414–419
24. ASBURY, A. J. (1986) Pupil response to alfentanil and fentanyl. A study in patients anaesthetised with halothane. *Anaesthesia*, **41**, 717–720
25. CULLEN, D. J., EGER, E. I., STEVENS, W. C., SMITH, N. T., CROMWELL, T. H., CULLEN, B. F. *et al.* (1972) Clinical signs of anesthesia. *Anesthesiology*, **36**, 21–36
26. COAKLEY, D., THOMAS, J. G. and LUNN, J. N. (1976) The effect of anaesthesia on ocular microtremor. *British Journal of Anaesthesia*, **48**, 1122–1123
27. TASHIRO, C., MURANISHI, R., GOMYO, I., MASHIMO, T. and YOSHIYA, I. (1983) Electroretinogram; a possible monitoring to brain hypoxia and anesthetic depth. *Anesthesiology*, **59**, A390
28. FLAGG, P. J. (1944) *The Art of Anaesthesia*, p. 105. London: J. B. Lippincott
29. GODDARD, G. F. (1982) A pilot study of changes in skin electrical conductance in patients undergoing general anaesthesia and surgery. *Anaesthesia*, **37**, 408–415

30. MARYNIAK, J. K. and BISHOP, V. A. (1987) Palmar sweat and heart rate changes during stress response attenuation with alfentanil. *British Journal of Anaesthesia*, **59**, 133P

31. NISHINO, T., HONDA, Y., KOHCHI, T., SHIRAHATA, M. and YONEZAWA, T. (1985) Effects of increasing depth of anaesthesia on phrenic nerve and hypoglossal nerve activity during the swallowing reflex in cats. *British Journal of Anaesthesia*, **57**, 208–213

32. WEIDRINGER, J. W. (1982) Bowel sound recording for gastrointestinal motility. In *Motility of the Digestive Tract*, edited by M. Weirbeck, pp. 273–278. New York: Raven Press

33. TUNSTALL, M. E. (1977) Detecting wakefulness during general anaesthesia for caesarean section. *British Medical Journal*, **1**, 1321

34. RUSSEL, I. F. (1986) Comparison of wakefulness with two anaesthetic regimens. Total i.v. v. balanced anaesthesia. *British Journal of Anaesthesia*, **58**, 965–968

Chapter 5

The EEG and detection of responsiveness during anaesthesia and coma

Pamela F. Prior

Patients or their relatives and doctors may question whether an unconscious person is aware of pain or sounds. Is a comatose child unaffected by the voice of its parent? Will an anaesthetic really ensure the desired oblivion during painful surgery? It seems natural to turn to the patient's brain for some form of answer, for some gauge of the depth of unconsciousness and for some evidence of responsiveness to external events. Neurophysiological techniques, such as recording the electroencephalogram (EEG) or the potentials evoked by specific sensory stimuli, allow us to do this. Traditionally such appraisal has been undertaken with the EEG, often displayed together with measurements of motor and autonomic functions such as the electromyogram (EMG) and the heart (from the electrocardiogram, ECG) and respiratory rates. The greatest clinical value of these techniques has been in the detection of responsiveness in patients unable to respond verbally or by movement because of physical limitations, coma, or drugs such as muscle relaxants, major sedatives or anaesthetics.

The brain, in common with the heart, nerves and muscles, generates spontaneous electrical potentials as a product of cellular metabolism. These small potentials can be recorded externally, for the EEG, by means of electrodes attached to the scalp. The electrical activity is closely related to brain function and its waveforms vary considerably with the state of the individual. Thus a patient who is deeply unconscious has a completely different EEG pattern to one who is lightly asleep or to one who is wide awake. A key difference between three such individuals will be their responses to noises or pain.

Auditory and painful stimuli activate extremely brief, specific potentials (the evoked or event-related potentials) which can be detected non-invasively from the peripheral nerve, brainstem, thalamus and the cerebral cortex which they can reach within as little as one-hundredth of a second. The potentials recorded reflect the direct passage of the sensation along natural pathways. They are even smaller than the EEG, preceding, and presumably initiating, any longer-lasting, widespread cerebral (EEG) or somatic effects of the stimulus.

Sensory events also produce general effects on the whole body. These are mediated by the brain through the autonomic nervous system, their extent and duration being related to the nature of the stimulus and the state of the individual. This is exemplified by the extreme bodily reaction to a frightening noise in the night, but the ability to sleep apparently undisturbed in a familiar noisy environment or when obtunded by drugs or stupor. Much of our understanding of the arousal mechanisms concerned is based upon observations from experimental recordings which have permitted observation of neuronal activity in cortical, subcortical, brainstem and autonomic pathways as well as the effects on the cardiovascular, respiratory and other systems.

It is impossible to know with certainty in an unconscious patient whether these general cerebral or autonomic responses, or even the modality-specific sensory evoked potentials, indicate conscious perception of pain or sounds. However, even though the alterations in autonomic functions may occur entirely at a subcortical or reflex level, it has to be assumed that any change in the functional activity of the cerebral cortex is an indication that the patient *might* be aware of the causative event. EEG alterations in response to pain provide reasonable evidence that anaesthesia or coma may be very 'light' and that the patient *may* subsequently recall the events.

This chapter begins with a brief outline of the nature of the EEG and the basic recording methods used for clinical monitoring. This account is followed by an indication of the types of alteration occurring at different depths of anaesthesia or coma, and a description of the type of EEG changes to be expected when a sensory stimulus such as pain or sound affects the brain.

The EEG

Basic mechanisms

Brain cellular oxidative metabolism leads to the electrochemical changes which are the basis of neural function. Neurones have a high concentration of potassium ions (K^+) and a low concentration of sodium ions (Na^+) in comparison with extracellular fluid. This concentration gradient is maintained by the sodium–potassium pump which exchanges intracellular Na^+ ions for extracellular K^+ ions. The resting membrane has a high permeability for K^+ which diffuses out of the neurone, but this is opposed by an electrical gradient of 70 mV (negative inside the cell) across the membrane created by the diffusion. This electrical gradient is reversed during an action potential and the inside of the neurone becomes about 30 mV positive compared with the outside, because there is a transient increase in the membrane's permeability to Na^+ when it is depolarized to a certain threshold. The membrane then repolarizes to its original value due to inactivation of Na^+ channels and an increase in K^+ permeability. The action potential, once started, is self-propagating without decrement along the axon to its terminal synapses with the bodies or dendrites of other neurones. After chemical transmission across the synapses, inhibitory (more negative) or excitatory (more positive) postsynaptic potentials are triggered. When the summated effect of these postsynaptic potentials causes the membrane at an axon hillock to reach a threshold, a new action potential is triggered. It has been shown that groups of these summated postsynaptic potentials are synchronous with, and presumably causally related to, the negative and positive waves of the EEG[1].

Relationship between EEG and cerebral metabolism during anaesthesia and coma

The potentials recorded in the EEG bear a general relation to the level of cerebral blood flow and oxygen metabolism[2]. Thus, for example, a patient with high cortical metabolic activity during status epilepticus will show greater amounts of electrical activity in the EEG than a patient whose cortical metabolism is depressed by profound sedation or deep general anaesthesia. With deepening coma or general anaesthesia, there is a general slowing of the dominant frequency of the EEG and, ultimately, it becomes broken up by periods of electrical silence which sooner or later become total. Intermittent silent periods, separated by bursts of waves, are described by electroencephalographers as 'burst suppression' pattern and total electrical silence as an isoelectric or equipotential EEG. These two patterns occur when cerebral oxygen metabolism is depressed to the maximum possible by central nervous depressant drugs such as barbiturates[3]. Residual metabolic activity maintains cell viability and, when the serum levels of the drug fall, neuronal metabolism and the EEG can recover.

Responses to stimuli

Peripherally arising stimuli reach the brain by afferent systems which pass through the ascending reticular activating system of the brainstem[4]. There are both specific sensory systems dealing with intermittent events and non-specific ones dealing with continuous information about the state of the body. These ascending systems regulate the state of cerebral cortical metabolic function, and impose projected alterations on the innate EEG patterns. These changes are of three main types: desynchronization with appearance of 20–60 Hz fast rhythms (EEG activation), 6–10 Hz spindles and bursts of 1–3 Hz slow waves. These last are part of a selective response and depend on the nature and strength of the initiating stimulus[5]. This overall hierarchical control system can also lead to feedback of motor or autonomic responses which can initiate appropriate actions, or to control the internal homeostasis of the body. The mechanisms are reviewed by Lairy and Dell[6].

The normal moment-to-moment variability of many physical functions reflects these mechanisms for control of the organism in relation to its internal and external environment. Thus the beat-to-beat heart rate, the breathing, the arterial blood pressure, the skin blood flow, the intracranial pressure and the EEG may all show fluctuations on a time scale of the order of 1–6 per minute. These variations in physiological signals indicate normal responses and control mechanisms. They change in coma and may disappear in the presence of severe brain damage[7–12]. The variability of the EEG, often best seen in compressed tracings from EEG monitors, is a feature that is relevant in the assessment of depth of anaesthesia and responses to stimuli.

EEG versus evoked potentials in determination of arousal during anaesthesia

A reflection of the complex neural mechanisms which govern the response of the body to external events can be observed with the EEG or EEG–polygraphic recording. The specific passage of the initiating sensory input can be detected by the technique of averaged sensory evoked potentials. This is a newer clinical method, and is technically much more demanding than the EEG, not least because the potentials recorded are of about one-tenth the magnitude, being of the order of a few microvolts (μV), the EEG being in the range 10–100 μV and the ECG being measured in millivolts. Because the small evoked potentials have to be recognized in the much higher voltage scalp EEG, averaging techniques are needed to enhance the 'signal-to-noise' ratio. Often as many as 50–2000 or more stimuli have to be presented to the subject and their responses averaged before the potentials can be recognized and then plotted out. This takes several minutes for each run of averaging. Only with sequential moving average displays[13,14] is it really possible quickly to detect subtle or fluctuating alterations in the patient's state.

The brainstem components of the auditory and somatosensory evoked potentials can be detected even during very deep anaesthesia or overdose with barbiturates and certain intravenous anaesthetic agents. They may persist even when the cortical components of the evoked potential and the EEG itself are markedly depressed or even extinguished. This has certain advantages in assessment of comatose or anaesthetized patients. However, the short-latency brainstem and primary cortical potentials by themselves do not necessarily indicate that the patient has been affected by a stimulus in the way that an EEG arousal response and accompanying autonomic changes may suggest. More details of the use of the brainstem auditory evoked potentials in increasing our understanding of mechanisms of anaesthesia[15] are also given in Chapter 12.

EEG methodology for clinical monitoring

Recording techniques

The most difficult part of EEG or evoked potential monitoring is the recording technique; professional help or advice cannot be recommended too strongly.

Appropriate scalp electrodes with low contact impedance are essential, and are usually chlorided silver EEG discs affixed to the scalp with collodion. In some circumstances, sterile intradermal needles may be suitable. Only a few (from two to six) electrodes are required for monitoring compared with over 20 for routine diagnostic EEGs in the laboratory. Optimal sites for the electrodes are those least likely to pick up unwanted potentials (artefacts) of biological or external origin. Bilateral centroparietal placements (positions C3–P3 and C4–P4 of the 10:20 system of the International Federation of Societies for Electroencephalography and Clinical Neurophysiology[16]) are preferable to those including frontal or temporal electrode placements, because of the lesser risk of picking up slow waves due to eye movements or sweating and faster components from scalp or facial musculature. Good recording technique is especially important when using special monitoring systems that do not allow visualization of the raw EEG to ensure that there is no contamination of the recording by artefact.

Data reduction, analysis and display

It is usually necessary, because of the voluminous and complex nature of conventional paper chart EEG recordings, to use a specially designed EEG monitoring system. Such systems analyse the EEG to display chosen features of interest, usually in a compressed and easily understandable form. They also incorporate techniques to help reduce contamination by the various extraneous signals which can give rise to such difficulties during EEG recording in the operating room or intensive care unit.

Choice of an appropriate type of EEG monitor can be difficult now that so many different systems are appearing on the market. Traditionally, there have been two main types. One gives a continuous display of changing EEG voltage with time, such as that of the EEG integrator of Drohocki and Drohocka[17] or the cerebral function monitor (CFM)[18]. The other type uses EEG frequency analysis obtained by either electronic filtering, by counts of baseline (0 µV) crossing by the EEG waves, or by Fourier analysis[19]. The results are displayed by sequential linear plots (smoothed histograms) of EEG frequency content, updated at regular intervals, as in the compressed spectral array (CSA)[20]. Both systems have some limitations. The new generation of EEG monitors[21–24] usually combine the best of both and deploy continuous voltage with averaged (over very short epochs of time) frequency displays. The latter are sometimes highlighted with markers of asymmetries or of the median spectral frequency[25] or the so-called spectral edge frequency[26]. These modern EEG monitors generally incorporate facilities for displaying the unprocessed EEG and for deriving quantitative data. The basic principles involved in the equipment and in making an informed choice, as well as a review of comparative studies, are given by Prior and Maynard[27].

EEG alterations with general anaesthesia

It has already been mentioned that, as coma or anaesthesia deepen, a series of superficially similar EEG changes occur fairly uniformly over the brain[28–32]. If the sequential alterations following induction of anaesthesia from the unpremedicated resting state are examined, it is evident that the pattern alterations are more complex than a simple reduction of frequency which progresses eventually to burst suppression pattern and electrical silence. There are complex changes with induction which start with an initial increase in fast components, especially with the rapidly acting intravenous anaesthetic agents. Amplitude increases and a variable admixture of slower frequencies then appears. The slow components then increase such that the dominant or median frequency gradually falls as anaesthesia deepens through a moderate range. Burst suppression pattern heralds deep anaesthesia and, during its bursts, a wide range of frequencies, including fast components, may still be represented. Thus both induction and deep anaesthesia are associated with complex EEG patterns, even though the intervening phases show simpler, more easily quantified, alterations.

There are considerable differences between agents within the same general EEG patterns[33], at least in part related to their rate of delivery to the brain, e.g. whether administered by inhalation or intravenously, and to different metabolic patterns in different individuals[34].

Correlations between EEG features and blood concentration of anaesthetic

Martin, Faulconer and Bickford[35] plotted arbitrary levels of integrated EEG amplitude against arterial concentration, which demonstrated linear relationships during moderate levels of anaesthesia. Between the late 1940s and the 1960s there were many efforts to produce automatic servocontrol of anaesthesia using EEG systems based upon feedback of integrated amplitude[36]. Since that time, the introduction of balanced combinations of neuromuscular and pain blockade with sleep doses of general anaesthetics has rendered such simple servocontrol systems obsolete. It is only with the desire for precise control of intravenous infusion anaesthesia that neurophysiological feedback loops have again become topical.

More recently, there have been a number of elegant studies, most of which examine the effects of sequential intravenous bolus doses, in which various single EEG measures have been shown to be correlated highly with serum levels of the single anaesthetic agent used[37–42]. These relationships are restricted to observations during light to moderate depths of anaesthesia produced by a single agent; the reported relationships tend to be more complex or break down during induction or deep anaesthesia[43], and when combinations of different agents are used[33]. Nonetheless, this work shows that, during clinically relevant depths of anaesthesia, simple measures based upon the EEG can be used to predict the depth of anaesthesia and, therefore, whether it is likely to be adequate for a particular patient.

Arousal patterns in the EEG

The key to more absolute understanding that one particular individual is awake or aroused by an external event is not prediction based on the behaviour of the average 'man on the Clapham omnibus'. Different patients handle their anaesthetics differently, different degrees of pain blockade may have been provided and the different degrees of pain inherent in different types of surgery will all add up to considerable inter-individual variations in the adequacy of a routine anaesthetic.

Careful monitoring for recognition of signs suggestive of pain or sounds which cause arousal in a particular patient, is more likely to enable us to recognize the unexpected. The observant anaesthetist has traditionally used several clinical signs for this purpose; unfortunately, with modern techniques they may not always be available to him. The EEG signs of arousal are well known from the recordings in drowsy, sleeping, stuporose and comatose subjects, and from those of patients who are inadequately sedated or anaesthetized. The EEG evidence is generally very simple and easily learned: it consists of *abrupt and quite marked change in the overall pattern of the recording*. When correctly identified and confirmed by observation of the effect of a second judiciously applied stimulus, the EEG changes provide unambiguous evidence that specific events have caused abrupt alterations in the functional state of the cerebral cortex.

Arousal during coma

The nature of these responses to stimuli varies according to the previous state of the subject, as mentioned in the review of basic mechanisms of the EEG. Thus, the effect of extraneous noise is different in the waking state and in drowsiness and light sleep. The awake subject, resting quietly or even drowsy with the eyes closed, exhibits a reduction in rhythmic EEG activities in response to a voice (the attenuation of the alpha rhythm so regularly tested in diagnostic recordings). In a drowsier or sleeping subject, there may be either an abrupt return to a waking pattern or a transient phenomenon, the K-complex, lasting about one second (*Figure 5.1*). If the subject has an abnormally functioning brain, there may commonly be a much more exaggerated pattern of arousal in the EEG (*Figure 5.2*), which consists of a more or less prolonged burst of high voltage slow waves[5,7,8,44,45]. These abnormal responses are common to many types of coma and provide useful information during the intensive care of unconscious patients. They can alert staff to the possibility that the patient is hearing conversations or feeling pain. They can also indicate whether sensory stimuli, applied to each limb separately, produce cerebral effects, demonstrating that a patient in post-traumatic coma has some degree of integrity of peripheral and central somatosensory

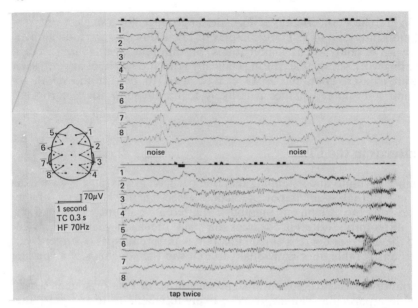

Figure 5.1 Two samples from a conventional EEG recording during natural sleep in a 26-year-old man to show intermittent (upper sample) and sustained (lower sample) alterations produced by auditory stimuli. In the upper sample during light (stage 2) sleep, high voltage K-complexes are initiated on two occasions following noises outside the recording suite. In the lower sample, during slightly lighter stage 2 sleep, the technician tapped her pencil on the EEG machine and elicited an immediate return to a waking EEG and, 8 seconds later, a burst of scalp muscle potentials and a movement artefact

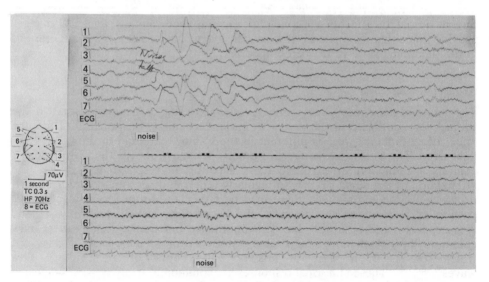

Figure 5.2 Arousal patterns in a 24-year-old man suffering from heat stroke and water intoxication. In the upper sample, recorded in the intensive care unit while he was in light coma, two nurses talking near his bed led to a high voltage slow wave response in the EEG with an initial increase, then a decrease in heart rate. A degraded K-complex is evident on the right. In the lower sample, recorded 4 days later when the patient had regained consciousness, but was not fully orientated, noises led to much lesser events in the EEG

pathways. This can help with diagnosis and prognostication, especially when neurological examination is impaired by muscle relaxants or injured limbs.

Arousal during anaesthesia

The anaesthetist needs to have precise and direct non-invasive information concerning the functional state of the brain to enable him to know when a particular patient is likely to be at risk of arousal responses or awakenings. To provide this we must focus our attention upon what actually happens when a patient rouses or wakes during anaesthesia and the detection of signs in the EEG[27] or other physiological monitors that warn when this is likely to happen. The conscious brain is characterized by reactivity to external environmental stimuli. It produces a rich variety of abruptly changing brain and EEG response patterns, the most gross being associated with autonomic and motor concomitants. They are similar in general terms to those seen during coma and consist of either sustained changes in the pattern (voltage, frequency or variability of the EEG, *see Figure 5.3*) or abrupt changes which last for a few seconds or minutes (*Figure 5.4*). They start abruptly following a sensory stimulus and may be reversed by supplementary doses of anaesthetic. If these latter lead to EEG alterations comparable to those during induction of anaesthesia, it is a strong indication that the patient was indeed virtually awake.

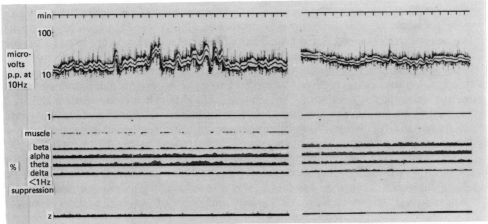

Figure 5.3 Two samples from EEG monitor recordings made with the cerebral function analysing monitor (CFAM) (for details *see* Chapter 8). On the left a 30-year-old man is drowsing spontaneously and being roused intermittently by people talking and moving equipment near to him. On the right a 37-year-old woman is very lightly anaesthetized (after thiopentone 5 mg/kg induction, administration of 0.5% isoflurane had just begun). Contrast the marked variability in amplitude and in the percentage frequency content and the presence of scalp muscle potentials (EMG) on the left with the much lesser (but still apparent) EEG variability and the absence of scalp muscle potentials on the right

Whether such EEG responses propagated via the brainstem reticular activating system and thalamus to the cerebral cortex represent conscious appreciation of surgical stimuli is another question altogether. There seems little doubt, however, that cerebral oxygen metabolism and blood flow, sympathetic activity and stress responses increase at the time of EEG arousal responses, even if the patient does not subsequently recall the causative stimulus. The arousal responses can be readily

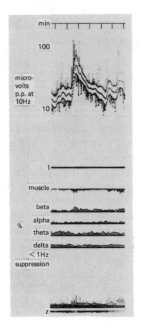

Figure 5.4 EEG monitored with the CFAM (for details *see* Chapter 8) during spontaneous drowsiness in a 50-year-old woman to show the pronounced effect of a loud auditory stimulus. The easily recognizable amplitude increase (upper part of the trace) is of abrupt onset and persisted for 3–4 minutes. Scalp muscle potentials also increase and the percentage of faster (beta) components rises at the expense of that of the slower (theta and delta) ones

identified visually in the conventional EEG recording and with any of the EEG monitors that provide a continuous display of voltage or amplitude including its variability (*see Figures 5.3* and *5.4*). They cannot presently be categorized by simple univariate EEG monitors using measures of analysis such as alteration in mean frequency. For high technology automatic warning systems, some form of pattern recognition process is required – something that the experienced human observer is better at than the computer. The methods might well include both EEG and non-EEG variables such as scalp muscle potentials or cardiac (absolute heart rate or its variability) changes[46]. Pattern recognition techniques have proved powerful tools in medicine and have been successfully applied to the EEG after cardiac arrest and in epilepsy monitoring systems[47–49]. It seems likely that profiles for different anaesthetic procedures can be derived that will allow deviations to be highlighted to generate automatic warning systems for clinical monitoring. Alternatively, the much lower technology approach, of watching an EEG monitor for simple pattern changes, has much to commend it.

Conclusion

The development and widespread introduction of appropriately designed neurophysiological monitoring systems to help ensure that patients were adequately anaesthetized would have practical value in improving quality of clinical care. The training of junior staff would be enhanced by feedback of performance in the same way that a young neurosurgeon learns when traction on a nerve is too great from audiofeedback of an evoked potential. From a medicolegal point of view, some form of permanent objective neurophysiological documentation of the adequacy of anaesthetic depth can advantageously be combined with the traditional handwritten anaesthetic chart in the patient's case notes.

Acknowledgements

A. R. Lloyd-Thomas, D. E. Maynard, T. M. Savege and S. B. Stefansson are thanked for the help they have given in forming the ideas presented here, but the author bears responsibility for any misinterpretation of their views.

References

1. CREUTZFELD, O. D., WATANABE, S. and LUX, A. D. (1966) Relations between EEG phenomena and potentials of single cortical cells. II Spontaneous and convulsive activity. *Electroencephalography and Clinical Neurophysiology,* **20,** 19–37

2. SULG, I. A., SOTANIEMI, K. A., TOLONEN, U. and KOKKANEN, E. (1981) Dependence between cerebral metabolism and blood flow as reflected in quantitative EEG. A critical review. *Advances in Biological Psychiatry,* **6,** 102–108

3. MICHENFELDER, J. D. (1974) The interdependency of cerebral functional and metabolic effects following massive doses of thiopental in the dog. *Anesthesiology,* **41,** 231–236

4. MORUZZI, G. and MAGOUN, H. W. (1949) Brain stem reticular formation and activation of the EEG. *Electroencephalography and Clinical Neurophysiology,* **1,** 455–473

5. KAADA, B. R., THOMAS, G., ALNAES, E. and WESTER, K. (1967) EEG synchronisation induced by high frequency midbrain reticular stimulation in anaesthetised cats. *Electroencephalography and Clinical Neurophysiology,* **22,** 220–230

6. LAIRY, G. C. and DELL, P. (1957) La régulation de l'activité corticale: aspects psychologiques et psychopathologiques. In *Conditionnement et Réactivite en Électroencéphalographie,* edited by H. Fischgold and H. Gastaut, *Electroencephalography and Clinical Neurophysiology,* Suppl. 6. Paris: Masson et Cie

7. EVANS, B. M. (1975) Cyclic changes in subacute spongiform and anoxic encephalopathy. *Electroencephalography and Clinical Neurophysiology,* **39,** 587–598

8. EVANS, B. M. (1976) Patterns of arousal in comatose patients. *Journal of Neurology, Neurosurgery and Psychiatry,* **39,** 392–402

9. BRICOLO, A., TURAZZI, F., FACCIOLI, F., ODORIZZI, F., SCIARETTA, G. and ERCULIANI, P. (1978) Clinical applications of compressed spectral array in long-term EEG monitoring of comatose patients. *Elecroencephalography and Clinical Neurophysiology,* **45,** 211–225

10. BRICOLO, A., FACCIOLI, F. and TURAZZI, F. (1979) L'EEG dans le coma traumatique aigu valeur diagnostique et pronostique. *Revue de EEG et Neurophysiologie Clinique,* **9,** 116–130

11. KARNAZE, D. S., MARSHALL, L. F. and BICKFORD, R. G. (1982) EEG monitoring of clinical coma: the compressed spectral array. *Neurology,* **32,** 289–292

12. MORILLO, L. E., TULLOCH, J. W., GUMNIT, R. J. and SNYDER, B. D. (1982) Compressed spectral array patterns following cardiopulmonary arrest. *Archives of Neurology,* **40,** 287–289

13. PFURTSCHELLER, G. (1986) Monitoring of spontaneous and evoked brain activity. In *Abstracts I, VIIth European Congress of Anaesthesiology,* edited by H. Bergman, K. Kramer and K. Steinbereithner), *Beitrage zur Anesthesiologie und Intensivmedizin,* **16,** 268–269

14. BERTRAND, O., GARCIA-LARREA, L., PERNIER, F., MAUGUIÈRE, F. and ARTRU, F. (1987) Brain-stem monitoring I. A system for high-rate sequential BAEP recording and feature extraction. *Electroencephalography and Clinical Neurophysiology,* (in press)

15. JONES, J. G. and KONIECZKO, K. (1986) Hearing and memory loss in anaesthetised patients. *British Medical Journal,* **292,** 1291–1293

16. INTERNATIONAL FEDERATION OF SOCIETIES FOR ELECTROENCEPHALOGRAPHY AND CLINICAL NEUROPHYSIOL-OGY (1983) *Recommendations for the Practice of Clinical Neurophysiology.* Amsterdam: Elsevier

17. DROHOCKI, Z. and DROHOCKA, J. (1939) L'électrospectrogramme du cerveau. *Comptes rendus des Séances de la Société de Biologie, Paris,* **130,** 95–98; DROHOCKI, Z. and DROHOKA, J. (1939) L'electrospectrographie quantitative du cerveau a l'etat de vielle et pendant la narcose. *Comptes rendus des Séances de la Société de Biologie, Paris,* **132,** 494–498

18. MAYNARD, D., PRIOR, P. F. and SCOTT, D. F. (1969) Device for continuous monitoring of cerebral activity in resuscitated patients. *British Medical Journal,* **4,** 545–546

19. DIETSCH, G. (1932) Fourier-analyse von Elektroencephalogrammen des Menschen. *Pflüger's Archiv für gesamte Physiologie des Menschen und der Tiere*, **230**, 106–112
20. BICKFORD, R. G., BILLINGER, T. W., SIMS, J., STEWARD, L. and HOFFMAN, R. (1973) Compressed spectral array in clinical EEG. In *Automation of Clinical Electroencephalography*, edited by P. Kellaway and I. Petersén, pp. 55–64. New York: Raven Press
21. MAYNARD, D. E. (1977) The cerebral function analyser monitor (CFAM). *Electroencephalography and Clinical Neurophysiology*, **43**, 479P
22. KLEIN, F. F. and DAVIS, D. A. (1981) A further statement on automated EEG processing for intraoperative monitoring. *Anesthesiology*, **54**, 433–434
23. PRONK, R. A. F. (1986) Peri-operative monitoring. In *Clinical Applications of Computer Analysis of EEG and other Neurophysiological signals*, edited by F. H. Lopes da Silva, W. Strom van Leeuwen and A. Rémond. *Handbook of Electroencephalography and Clinical Neurophysiology*, revised series, Vol. 2, pp. 93–130. Amsterdam: Elsevier
24. MAYNARD, D. E. and JENKINSON, J. L. (1984) The cerebral function analysing monitor. Initial clinical experience, application and further development. *Anaesthesia*, **39**, 678–690
25. STOECKEL, H., SCHWILDEN, H., LAUVEN, P. and SCHÜTTLER, J. (1981) EEG parameters for evaluation of depth of anaesthesia. In *Proceedings of the European Academy of Anaesthesiology*, edited by M. D. Vickers and J. Crul, pp. 73–84. Berlin: Springer Verlag
26. RAMPIL, I. J., HOLZER, J. A., QUEST, D. O., ROSENBAUM, S. H. and CORRELL, J. W. (1983) Prognostic value of computerized EEG analysis during carotid endarterectomy. *Anesthesia and Analgesia*, **62**, 186–192
27. PRIOR, P. F. and MAYNARD, D. E. (1986) *Monitoring Cerebral Function*, 2nd edn. Amsterdam: Elsevier Biomedical Press
28. ROMANO, J. and ENGEL, G. L. (1944) Delirium. I. EEG patterns. *Archives of Neurology and Psychiatry (Chicago)*, **51**, 356–377
29. COURTIN, R. F., BICKFORD, R. G. and FAULCONER, A. JR (1950) Classification and significance of electro-encephalographic patterns produced by nitrous-oxide-ether anesthesia during surgical operations. *Proceedings of the Staff Meetings of the Mayo Clinic*, **25**, 197–206
30. FAULCONER, A. JR and BICKFORD, R. G. (1960) *Electroencephalography in Anesthesiology*. Springfield, Illinois: Thomas
31. CLARK, D. L. and ROSNER, B. S. (1973) Neurophysiologic effects of general anesthetics: I. The electroencephalogram and sensory evoked potentials in man. *Anesthesiology*, **38**, 564–582
32. ROSNER, B. S. and CLARK, D. L. (1973) Neurophysiologic effects of general anesthetics. II. Sequential regional actions in the brain. *Anesthesiology*, **39**, 59–81
33. PICHLMAYR, I., LIPS, U. and KUNKEL, H. (1984) *The Electroencephalogram in Anaesthesia. Fundamentals, Practical Applications, Examples*. Berlin: Springer-Verlag
34. HORNER, T. D. and STANSKI, D. R. (1985) The effect of increasing age on thiopental disposition and anesthetic requirement. *Anesthesiology*, **62**, 714–724
35. MARTIN, J. T., FAULCONER, A. and BICKFORD, R. G. (1959) Electroencephalography in anesthesiology. *Anesthesiology*, **20**, 359–376
36. BICKFORD, R. G. (1949) Neurophysiological applications of an automatic anesthetic regulator controlled by brain potentials. *American Journal of Physiology*, **159**, 562–563
37. DOENICKE, A., LOEFFLER, B., KUGLER, J., SUFFMANN, H. and GROTE, B. (1982) Plasma concentrations and EEG after various regimens of etomidate. *British Journal of Anaesthesia*, **54**, 393–400
38. FRANK, M., SAVEGE, T. M., LEIGH, J., GREENWOOD, J. and HOLLY, J. M. P. (1982) Comparison of the cerebral function monitor and plasma concentrations of thiopentone and alphaxalone during total i.v. anaesthesia with repeated bolus doses of thiopentone and althesin. *British Journal of Anaesthesia*, **54**, 609–616
39. FRANK, M., MAYNARD, D. E., TSANICLIS, L. M., MAJOR, E. and COUTINO, P. E. (1984) Changes in cerebral electrical activity measured by the cerebral function analysing monitor following bolus injections of thiopentone. *British Journal of Anaesthesia*, **56**, 1075–1081
40. HUDSON, R. J., STANSKI, D. R., SAIDMAN, L. J. and MEATHE, E. (1983) A model for studying depth of anesthesia and acute tolerance to thiopental. *Anesthesiology*, **59**, 301–308

41. SCHWILDEN, H., SCHÜTTLER, J. and STOECKEL, H. (1985) Quantitation of the EEG and pharmacodynamic modelling of hypnotic drugs: etomidate as an example. *European Journal of Anaesthesiology,* **2,** 121–131

42. SCHÜTTLER, J., SCHWILDEN, H. and STOECKEL, H. (1985) Infusion strategies to investigate the pharmacokinetics and pharmacodynamics of hypnotic drugs: etomidate as an example. *European Journal of Anaesthesiology,* **2,** 133–142

43. LEVY, W. A. (1984) Intraoperative EEG patterns: implications for EEG monitoring. *Anesthesiology,* **60,** 430–434

44. SCHWARTZ, M. S. and SCOTT, D. F. (1978) Pathological stimulus-related slow wave arousal responses in the EEG. *Acta Neurologica Scandinavica,* **57,** 300–304

45. KAADA, B. R., HARKMARK, W. and STOKKE, O. (1961) Deep coma associated with desynchronization in the EEG. *Electroencephalography and Clinical Neurophysiology,* **13,** 785–789

46. INTERNATIONAL FEDERATION OF SOCIETIES FOR ELECTROENCEPHALOGRAPHY AND CLINICAL NEUROPHYSIOL-OGY (1987) The methodology of recording non-EEG physiological variables ('polygraphy') in association with EEG and standards of practice in EEG polygraphy. In *Recommendations for the Practice of Clinical Neurophysiology,* Vol. 2, edited by R. J. Ellingson and D. W. Class. Amsterdam: Elsevier (in press)

47. BINNIE, C. D., PRIOR, P. F., LLOYD, D. S. L., SCOTT, D. F. and MARGERISON, J. H. (1970) Electrocencephalographic prediction of fatal anoxic brain damage after resuscitation from cardiac arrest. *British Medical Journal,* **4,** 265–268

48. BINNIE, C. D. (1983) Telemetric EEG monitoring in epilepsy. In *Recent Advances in Epilepsy I,* edited by T. A. Pedley and B. S. Meldrum, pp. 155–178. Edinburgh: Churchill Livingstone

49. BINNIE, C. D. (1986) Computer applications in monitoring. In *Clinical Applications of Computer Analysis of EEG and other Neurophysiological Signals,* edited by F. H. Lopez da Silva, W. Strom van Leeuwen and A. Rémond. *Handbook of Electroencephalography and Clinical Neurophysiology,* revised series, Vol. 2, pp. 67–91. Amsterdam: Elsevier

Chapter 6

The unprocessed EEG

H. Schwilden and H. Stoeckel

Shortly after the first report on the recording of the electroencephalgram (EEG) in man by Berger[1] in 1929, it was recognized that this signal could be used to assess the neurophysiological or neuropathological state of the brain. A number of methods have been developed since to translate a given EEG tracing into a clinically meaningful statement.

Two approaches are used: the first technique of evaluation of the EEG is by *visual inspection* of recorded EEG epochs and subsequent staging of these epochs according to some classification (unprocessed EEG), for instance that of Rechtschaffen and Kales[2] for sleep staging. The second approach uses the principles of *random data analysis*[3], with the aim of data reduction and enhancement of the signal-to-noise ratio (processed EEG).

The widespread use of the latter approach was made possible by the availability of relatively affordable computer facilities. This had, however, led to an increase in so-called EEG trend-monitoring devices accompanied by an even greater number of EEG derivatives, generating numbers which are said to be useful in assessing changes in the EEG. The problems caused by the new devices are that any two publications which use different devices are not comparable and that any new method has to be used in hundreds of cases to achieve any correlation between the generated numbers and the clinical implications.

It thus becomes necessary carefully to investigate the properties and information of the unprocessed EEG and how certain EEG features may be manipulated or modified by signal processing techniques.

The 'unprocessed' EEG

EEG recording requires in general three elements: a set of electrodes, which are fixed at some location on the scalp; an amplifier, to amplify the current flowing between two electrodes; and an electromechanical device, to draw the corresponding EEG tracing.

The selection of each of these three elements influences the final EEG tracing, highlighting the point that even the 'unprocessed' EEG is a processed signal. The electrodes attached to the skin have not only an electrical resistance, but also a capacity, and therefore impedance, which itself modifies the frequency response. It is generally recommended that the electrical resistance measured at 10 Hz should be less than 5 kΩ. Mechanical inertia of the recording device adds additional distortion to the frequency. Hence a reasonably precise EEG recording is only possible in a frequency band, which is not affected by these mechanisms. Most EEG amplifiers are therefore equipped with two controls by which high and low frequency cut-off filters may be selected. The choice of these filters can be of utmost importance for the recording of the EEG during anaesthesia.

The range of low-frequency cut-off filters used in the anaesthetic literature ranges from 0.5 Hz[4] to 4 Hz[5]. The different filter settings may affect the EEG tracing considerably during anaesthesia, because up to 60% of total EEG activity can occur in the frequency range 0.5–2 Hz.

Two tracings of one EEG epoch filtered with two different low frequency cut-offs are shown in *Figure 6.1*. The upper trace refers to a filter setting of 0.5 Hz, the

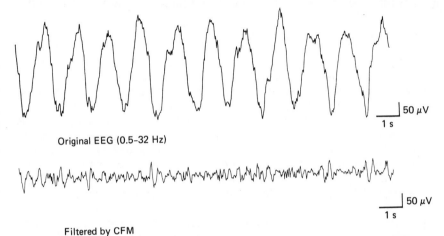

Original EEG (0.5-32 Hz)

Filtered by CFM

Figure 6.1 Different tracings of the same EEG epoch as obtained by different shapes of the filters. For the cerebral function monitor (CFM), it is assumed that the filter starts at 2 Hz[13]. (From Schwilden and Stoeckel[8])

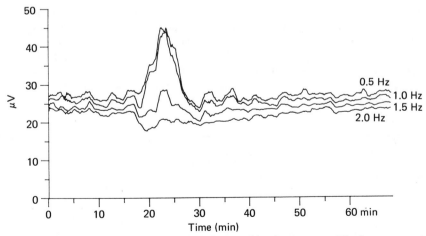

Figure 6.2 Time course of mean amplitude during carotid endarterectomy. The four curves refer to four different low frequency cut-offs at 0.5, 1, 1.5 and 2 Hz. If a high frequency cut-off is chosen, a reverse in trend can be observed; instead of increasing, mean amplitude decreases with a cut-off at 2 Hz. (From Schwilden and Stoeckel[8])

lower trace to a filter setting of 2 Hz. Both tracings are quire different and would suggest very different clinical stages. The upper drawing reflects a deep stage of anaesthesia, while the lower trace could be associated with a spontaneous beta-type baseline EEG or a barbiturate[6] or benzodiazepine[7] induced beta EEG during sedation or at very light planes of anaesthesia.

The implication of different filter settings for intra-operative trend monitoring is given on *Figure 6.2*. It compares the time course of mean amplitude of an EEG recorded during endarterectomy for four different low frequency cut-offs (0.5, 1, 1.5 and 2 Hz). The effect of the arterial clamping might be missed because of inappropriate selection of a filter.

Thus, even the so-called unprocessed EEG is a highly processed signal, because different EEG filter settings on the EEG machine generate quite different results.

The unprocessed EEG and anaesthesia-related EEG patterns

Power spectrum analysis assumes stationarity of the EEG signal. Distinct EEG patterns can violate this assumption. *Figure 6.3* depicts two EEG tracings during anaesthesia with enflurane and isoflurane which have two distinct patterns, burst suppression periods for both cases and also spike and wave patterns in the case of enflurane. The reason why patterns can violate the assumptions of stationarity is given in *Figure 6.4*. Analysis of an EEG epoch into sine waves of given frequencies, can result in plotting amplitudes and phases against the frequency, yielding the two graphs shown in the bottom part of *Figure 6.4*. The left-hand drawing gives a clear signal of maximum amplitude in the alpha band (8–13 Hz); the phases behave like white noise and, therefore, give no information. Consequently, for such periods the phases can be waived giving data reduction by a factor of two. In the case of distinct patterns, part of the information necessary to reconstruct the pattern is given by phase relationships[8]. Considerable misinterpretation is possible if the amplitudes (which are squared to give the power spectrum) are used by themselves. *Figure 6.5* depicts two power spectra in the lower part and the corresponding EEG tracings in the upper part.

While spike and wave complexes are said to be more specific for enflurane[9, 10], burst suppression can be observed with any anaesthetic agent. The frequency of their occurrence and their length depends on dosage. In a study with isoflurane, enflurane and halothane aiming at an alveolar concentration of 1.3 MAC ($n = 7$ for each agent) and 1.5 MAC ($n = 7$ for each agent) (where MAC = minimum alveolar concentration) in 60% nitrous oxide, the frequency of occurrence of burst suppression observed during induction is shown in *Table 6.1*.

Table 6.1

Anaesthetic	Minimum alveolar concentration	Number of patients showing burst suppression
Isoflurane	1.5	7
	1.3	5
Enflurane	1.5	6
	1.3	2
Halothane	1.5	0
	1.3	0

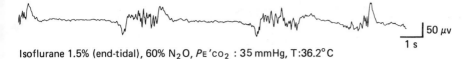

Isoflurane 1.5% (end-tidal), 60% N_2O, $PE'CO_2$: 35 mmHg, T:36.2°C

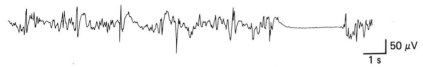

50 μV

1 s

Enflurane 2.1% (end-tidal), 60% N_2O, $PE'CO_2$: 34 mmHg, T:36.3°C

Figure 6.3 Typical EEG patterns, which violate the assumption of quasistationarity underlying power spectrum estimation, are spikes or spikes and waves during anaesthesia with enflurane, and burst suppression periods depicted for enflurane as well as isoflurane

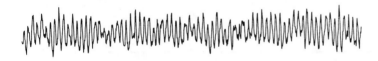

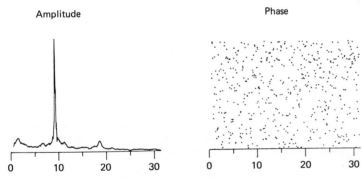

Amplitude

Phase

Figure 6.4 Decomposition of an alpha-type EEG into sinus waves, which are characterized by their amplitudes and phases. Plotting the amplitude and the phases against frequency results in a clear signal for the amplitude. The phases behave like white noise and can thus be omitted: this leads to data reduction by a factor of two. (From Schwilden and Stoeckel[8])

Automatic EEG processing and pattern recognition

Methods for estimating the power spectrum, such as Fourier analysis[11] or maximum entropy analysis[12], are rather sensitive in detecting even small frequency shifts of quasistationary signals, and are, therefore, in widespread use for EEG trend monitoring during anaesthesia. Relying, as they do, on the assumption of stationarity, they may, however, produce incorrect results if the signal is not tested for stationarity prior to power spectrum estimation. The most important violations

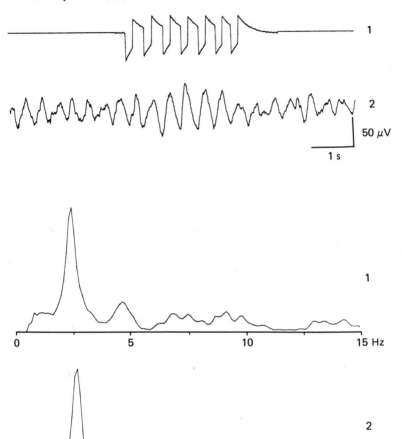

Figure 6.5 The power spectrum can give inadequate results if stationarity of the signal does not hold true. The rather similar power spectra (bottom part) belong to quite different EEG epochs (upper part). The first epoch depicts the gauging pattern of the EEG amplifier, the lower part the EEG of an anaesthetized individual

of stationarity within anaesthesia are by burst suppression pattern. Thus burst suppression must be properly recognized before further EEG processing can be reliable. An automatic pattern recognition procedure does, however, require a precise definition of a burst suppression rather than visual inspection of the EEG trace.

Obviously, a suppression period is given if the local amplitude of the EEG is decreased to a certain degree with respect to the deflections in the immediate neighbourhood. The authors investigated the question of how strongly and for what minimum time the mean amplitude has to be decreased, so that an automatic burst suppression pattern recognition algorithm would detect suppressions as identified by visual inspection. For this purpose, the EEG signal was sliced into intervals of 0.064 s. For each interval mean amplitude was calculated.

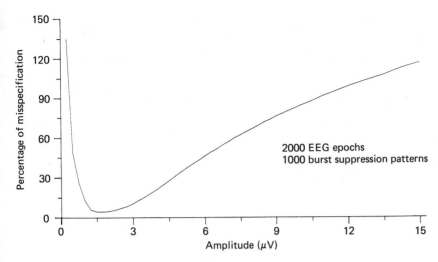

Figure 6.6 Automatic burst suppression pattern recognition requires a measure of amplitude, below which the suppression activity must occur, in order to match a visually identified suppression period. It was found that mean amplitude has to be in the order of 2 μV to minimize the percentage of misspecification between automatically recognized burst suppressions and visually recognized ones

It was observed that at least 10 adjacent epochs have to have a mean amplitude below a critical value in order to match the visually identified suppression periods. *Figure 6.6* shows the determination of the critical mean amplitude. For 1000 EEG epochs with visually identified burst suppressions out of a library of 2000 EEG epochs, it was estimated that mean amplitude must be below 2 μV so as to minimize the percentage of misspecification between automatic and visually recognized burst suppression pattern.

References

1. BERGER, H. (1929) Über das Elektroenkephalogrammm des Menschen I. *Archives of Psychiatry,* **87**, 527–570
2. RECHTSCHAFFEN, A. and KALES, A. (eds) (1968) *A Manual of Standardized Terminology, Techniques and Scoring System for Sleep Stages of Human Subjects.* US Department of Health, Education and Welfare. National Institute of Health, Bethesda, Maryland 20014. NIH Publication 204
3. BENDAT, J. S. and PIERSOL, A. G. (1971) *Random Data: Analysis and Measurement Procedures.* New York: Wiley Interscience
4. STOECKEL, H., SCHWILDEN, H., LAUVEN, P. and SCHÜTTLER, H. (1981) EEG parameters for evaluation of depth of anaesthesia: the median of frequency distribution. In *Proceedings of the European Academy of Anaesthesiology of 1980,* edited by M. D. Vickers and J. Crul. pp. 73–84. Berlin: Springer
5. LEVY, W. J., SHAPIRO, H. M., MARUCHACK, B. and MEATHE, E. (1980) Automatic EEG processing for intraoperative monitoring: a comparison of techniques. *Anesthiology,* **53**, 223–236
6. FAULCONER, A., JR and BICKFORD, R. G. (1960) *Electroencephalography in Medicine.* Springfield, Illinois: Thomas
7. FINK, M., IRWIN, P., WEINFIELD, R. E., SCHWARTZ, M. A. and CONNEY, A. H. (1976) Blood levels and electroencephalographic effects of diazepam and bromazepam. *Clinical Pharmacology and Therapeutics,* **20**, 184–191

8. SCHWILDEN, H. and STOECKEL, H. (1985) The derivation of EEG parameters for modelling and control of anaesthetic drug effect. In *Quantitation, Modelling and Control in Anaesthesia,* edited by H. Stoeckel, pp. 160–169. Stuttgart: Georg Thième

9. PERSSON, A., PETERSON, E. and WAHLIN, A. (1978) EEG-changes during general anaesthesia with enflurance (Efrane®) in comparison with ether. *Acta Anaesthesiologica Scandinavica,* **22,** 339–348

10. BURCHIEL, K. J., STOCKARD, J. J., CALVERLEY, R. K. and TY SMITH, N. (1977) Relationship of pre- and postanesthetic EEG abnormalities to enflurane-induced seizure activity. *Anesthesia and Analgesia,* **56,** 509–514

11. COOLEY, H. and TUCKEY, J. (1965) An algorithm for machine computation of complex Fourier series. *Mathetmatics of Computation,* **19,** 297–301

12. BURG, J. P. (1978) Maximum entropy spectral analysis. In *Modern Spectrum Analysis,* edited by D. G. Childers, pp. 34–41. New York: IEEE Press

13. PRIOR, P. F. (1979) *Monitoring Cerebral Function.* Amsterdam: Elsevier

Chapter 7

Median EEG frequency

H. Stoeckel and H. Schwilden

There seems to be no doubt that different anaesthetic agents can produce different EEG patterns. It is generally assumed that: EEG changes are directly related to biochemical changes each compound induces in the brain, and the behavioural effects are directly related to these biochemical effects[1]. The pharmaco-EEG[2,3] tries to identify a specific drug and its action on behaviour from its modifying actions on EEG patterns.

This chapter examines the problem of quantitation of the EEG effects of drugs used in anaesthesia, and the possible correlations to clinical aspects and signs. There are many drugs and many drug combinations used for general anaesthesia. How can derivatives of the EEG uniquely reflect their common therapeutic aim (analgesia and unconsciousness), without dependence upon the particular drugs or drug combinations used?

Spectral EEG derivations

The problem of estimating different degrees of consciousness (or unconsciousness) during anaesthesia by quantitative EEG analysis is that of constructing a description of a given EEG epoch by a number or set of numbers which can be shown to correlate with the depth of anaesthesia as estimated independently by clinical means. Ideally, this variable should be able to reflect trends and its actual value should allow for estimation of the plane of anaesthesia. Trend as well as parameter values should be independent of particular drugs and particular patients. Early work[4] showed that the frequency content of the EEG changes with depth of anaesthesia. This observation has established frequency analysis, Fourier analysis[5], as a valid tool in the investigation of changes in the EEG related to anaesthesia.

The power spectrum transforms a given EEG epoch into distribution of pure sine waves of varying frequencies which constitute the signal. The problem of developing spectral EEG parameters is thus identical to quantity distributions[6]. The classic approach to describe this distribution, i.e. the power spectrum, is the determination of the absolute or relative EEG power in the common clinically defined frequency bands[7]: delta, theta, alpha and beta bands. The power spectrum is thus transformed into a set of four numbers. The question has to be asked, however, whether these frequency bands represent an optimal or natural decomposition of the entire frequency range of the EEG[7]. These frequency bands represent a useful description and analysis of the EEG of the resting, awake subject[8], but it has been shown in recent years by factor analysis that the partition into frequency bands changes with depth of anaesthesia[9]. Hence the selection of a certain frequency band for monitoring during anaesthesia might be quite satisfactory at a given stage of consciousness, but might be inappropriate at other stages. Therefore, it has to be concluded that a suitable quantification of the EEG power spectrum should be independent of the frequency band structure. It is well known that, for normal distributions, the mean represents the most likely value. This is not true for multimodal distributions such as EEG power spectra. General statistics prove that the median of a distribution (50th quantile) is the most insensitive quantile with respect to outliers and represents best the measure of dispersion.

A power spectrum for clinical anaesthesia with enflurane in 60% nitrous oxide is shown in *Figure 7.1*. This case shows different stages of consciousness and

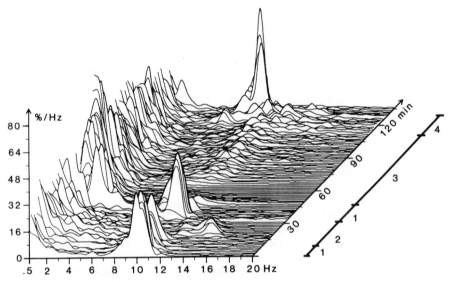

Figure 7.1 EEG power spectrum during clinical anaesthesia with enflurane in 60% nitrous oxide. Natural sleep and anaesthesia show similar EEG power spectra. (1) Awake; (2) sleep; (3) anaesthesia; (4) recovery

unconsciousness: the awake patient; natural not drug-induced sleep; sudden awakening followed by induction and maintenance of anaesthesia; and the recovery period. Natural sleep and anaesthesia may produce rather similar EEG patterns, as reflected in *Figure 7.1*, by similar EEG power spectra; these are clearly distinguished from the baseline EEG and the recovery period. The difference between sleep and anaesthesia is, however, characterized by the ability to wake up spontaneously or by acoustic stimuli during natural sleep, whereby anaesthesia tries to induce a state which is characterized by tolerance even to severe surgical stimuli.

Median EEG frequency

An indication that median EEG frequency is not only a mathematical abstraction, but might have some reasonable properties in relation to different levels of consciousness is given in *Figure 7.2*. This compares the time course of median frequency (lower part) with the time course of a visual staging of the EEG, as assessed by the prescription of Kugler[10], which for the depicted case was performed by Doenicke *et al.*[11]. It is quite obvious that median EEG frequency parallels the time course of the classification procedure, and both are closely related to the time course of the declining blood concentrations of etomidate. Assuming that higher concentrations are associated with deeper degrees of unconsciousness, this figure gives an example the deeper planes of anaesthesia are correlated to lower median values.

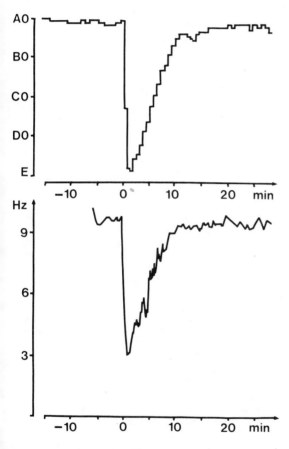

Figure 7.2 Comparison of the time course of median EEG frequency (lower trace) after an intravenous bolus of etomidate and staging of the produced EEG patterns (upper trace) according to the scheme of Kugler[10] as used by Doenicke *et al.*[11]

Intravenous hypnotics

The authors investigated the relationship between median EEG frequency, drug concentrations and apparent clinical signs more systematically. A study design consisted of three periods of infusion of etomidate to cause linearly increasing blood concentrations until the appearance of burst suppression, followed by an interval of no infusion until the volunteer recovered sufficiently to know where he was[12]. The time course of blood concentrations of etomidate and median EEG frequency for a typical volunteer is shown in *Figure 7.3*. The correlation of median

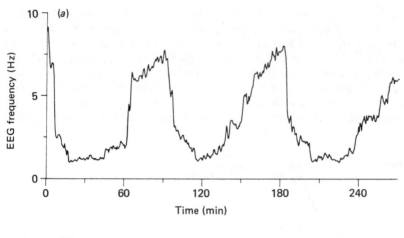

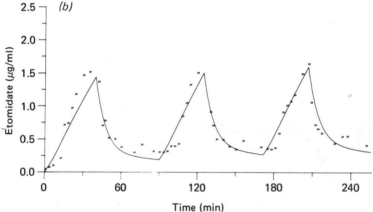

Figure 7.3 Time course of median EEG frequency (upper trace) during a three-fold repetitive infusion of etomidate, which produced linearly increasing etomidate concentrations (lower trace). The infusion was restarted if the subject had reached the level of orientation to time and place[13]. (*a*) Median frequency; (*b*) blood concentration of etomidate (measured versus predicted)

Table 7.1 Relationship between clinical signs and median EEG frequency in six volunteers during infusion of etomidate generating three times linearly increasing concentrations

Increase		Decrease	
Signs	*Median (Hz)**	*Median (Hz)**	*Signs*
Baseline (awake)	9.5 (0.4)	6.6 (0.6)	Full orientation
Falling asleep	4.8 (0.8)	4.7 (0.7)	Responsive
Corneal reflex Ø	2.0 (0.4)	2.0 (0.3)	Corneal reflex +
Burst suppression +	1.6 (0.3)	1.8 (0.3)	Burst suppression Ø

* Values in parentheses are the standard deviation.
Each cycle was commenced when the volunteer had reached proper personal orientation and was ceased if burst suppression on pattern occurred[6].

EEG frequency and clinical signs is given in *Table 7.1*. Induction of sleep occurred at median EEG frequency values of approximately 5 Hz and responsiveness was regained at nearly the same EEG level. Schüttler *et al.*[14] made similar observations in another study with ketamine and its isolated isomers (*Table 7.2*). It was not possible to reach a deeper plane of anaesthesia than excitation with the (−) ketamine isomer. Both *Tables 7.1* and *7.2* show that median values above 5 or 6 Hz might be associated with awareness.

Table 7.2 Relationship between clinical signs and median EEG frequency in six volunteers during infusion of ketamine and its enantiomers

Sign	Median frequency (Hz)*		
	(±)Ketamine	(+)Ketamine	(−)Ketamine
Baseline (awake)	9.5 (0.6)	9.9 (0.1)	9.8 (0.3)
Maximal effect	1.6 (0.9)	2.2 (0.9)	5.0 (0.6)
Responsive	6.3 (0.7)	5.7 (0.6)	6.1 (0.2)
Early orientation	7.1 (1.1)	6.3 (0.6)	6.4 (0.4)
Full orientation	7.8 (1.1)	7.2 (1.0)	7.1 (0.8)

* Values are: mean (standard deviation); $P<0.05$, (−)K versus (+)K and (−)K versus (±)K.
For the isomer (−)ketamine, it was not possible to induce a safe hypnotic effect[14].

Similar results were obtained during a closed-loop feedback control of methohexitone-induced anaesthesia. Thirteen volunteers were submitted to a model-based, adaptive, closed-loop feedback control of methohexitone infusion aimed at a median frequency of between 2 and 3 Hz for 2 hours[15]. None of the volunteers responded to commands when the median frequency was within this range. When the infusion was stopped the volunteers became responsive at a median value of 5.2 Hz on average, and were aware of time and place at 7.2 Hz. The median value for the latter stage was always higher than that at the time of responsiveness.

EEG slowing and, therefore, decrease in median frequency may, however, not follow drug concentrations. For thiopentone[16, 17] and propofol (unpublished data) at very low concentrations, high EEG frequencies can contribute considerably to the total EEG power and thus increase median EEG frequency; this decreases at higher concentrations of drug. The bell shape of the concentration–response curve can be interpreted in terms of different sensitivities of the inhibitory and excitatory neuronal systems of the brain[18, 17].

Volatile anaesthetics

A recent study with isoflurane at 1.3 and 1.5 MAC (where MAC is the minimum alveolar concentration at which 50% subjects react to a specified stimulus) in 60% nitrous oxide provided more evidence that awareness may occur at median EEG values above 5 Hz[19]. Two groups of seven patients were anaesthetized with isoflurane in 60% nitrous oxide at 1.3 and 1.5 MAC. Both groups had similar median values at baseline, during surgery and recovery. Time to recovery was approximately twice as long for the group treated with 1.5 MAC than for the group

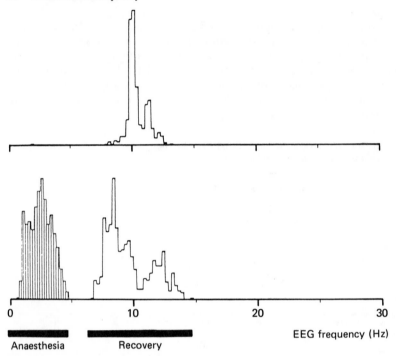

Figure 7.4 Distribution of median EEG frequency during anaesthesia with isoflurane in 60% nitrous oxide in 14 patients. The upper distribution represents median values as recorded awake (baseline). The bottom part compares the distributions during anaesthesia (left hand side) and recovery (after having responded to commands, right hand side)[19]

treated with 1.3 MAC. Both groups regained consciousness at a median value above 5 Hz. The merged distributions of median EEG frequency for both groups during baseline (upper part), anaesthesia and recovery are shown in *Figure 7.4*. In another study comparing the three volatile agents halothane, enflurane and isoflurane, it was observed that at drug concentrations of 1.3 MAC, or higher, median frequency was in general decreased to values at or below 5 Hz. *Figure 7.5* shows the percentages of EEG activity in the indicated frequency bands awake and during anaesthesia with halothane, enflurane and isoflurane in 60% nitrous oxide. For each drug a group of 14 patients was investigated.

Drug combinations

In a group of 35 patients, who were treated with a variety of drugs and drug combinations during clinical anaesthesia according to the discretion of the anaesthetist, 75% of all measured median frequencies were below 5 Hz (*Figure 7.6*)[21].

Thus, it has been shown that a wide variety of drugs used for general anaesthesia can be administered so that median EEG frequency is below 5 Hz. It has also been shown that median values above 5 Hz might be associated with responsiveness to verbal commands. It cannot be concluded from these findings that a median EEG frequency value below 5 Hz is necessary to avoid post-operative recall. However,

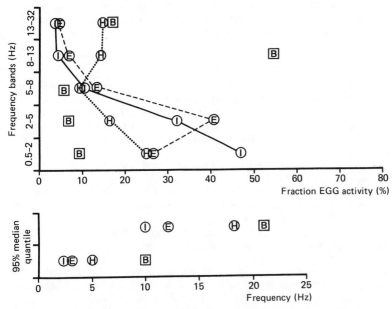

Figure 7.5 Spectral EEG parameters for halothane (H), enflurane (E) and isoflurane (I) at equipotent concentrations related to minimum alveolar concentration compared to baseline values (B). The upper drawing refers to the fraction of EEG activity in the indicated frequency bands. The lower part shows the results for the 95th quantile and median EEG frequency (50th quantile) of the EEG power spectrum[20]

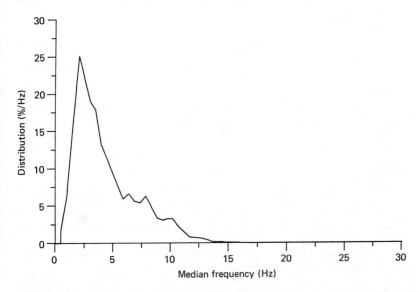

Figure 7.6 Distribution of median EEG frequency in 35 patients treated with a variety of drugs and drug combinations. Dosing was at the discretion of the anaesthetist[21]

making the assumption that post-operative recall has to be preceded by intra-operative awareness, it can be concluded that median values below 5 Hz reduce the likelihood of post-operative recall.

References

1. KÜNKEL, H. (1982) On hypotheses underlying pharmaco-electroencephalography. In *EEG in Drug Research*, edited by W. M. Herrmann, p. 1. Stuttgart: Gustav Fischer
2. DOLCE, G. and KÜNKEL, H. (1975) *CEAN – Computerized EEG Analysis*. Stuttgart: Gustav Fischer
3. HERRMANN, W. M. (1982) *Electroencephalography in Drug Research*. Stuttgart: Gustav Fischer
4. FAULCONER, A. and BICKFORD, R. G. (1960) *Electroencephalography in Anesthesiology*. Springfield, Illinois: C. Thomas
5. COOLEY, H. and TUCKEY, J. (1965) An algorithm for machine computation of complex Fourier series. *Mathematics of Computation*, **19**, 297–301
6. SCHWILDEN, H. and STOECKEL, H. (1985) The derivation of EEG parameters for modelling and control of anaesthetic drug effect. In *Quantitation, Modelling and Control in Anaesthesia*, edited by H. Stoeckel, pp. 160–169. Stuttgart: Georg Thième
7. MATEJCEK, M. (1982) Vigilance and the EEG: Psychological, physiological and pharmacological aspects. In *EEG in Drug Research*, edited by W. M. Hermann, pp. 405–508. Stuttgart: Gustav Fischer
8. HERRMAN, W. M., FICHTE, K. and KUBICKI, ST. (1980) Definition von EEG-Frequenzbändern aufgrund strukturanalytischer Betrachtungen. In *Factor Analysis and EEG variables*, edited by St. Kubicki, W. M. Herrmann and G. Laudahn, pp. 61–88. Stuttgart: Gustav Fischer
9. SCHWILDEN, H. and STOECKEL, H. (1981) Faktorenanalyse der Frequenzbandverteilung des EEG während Halothan- und Enflurannarkose. In *Inhalationsanästhesie-heute und morgen. Anästhesiologie und Notfallmediazin*, edited by K. Peter and F. Jesche, Vol. 149, pp. 143–152. Berlin: Springer
10. KUGLER, J. (1966) *Elektroencephalographie in Klinik und Praxis*, 2nd edn. Stuttgart: Thième
11. DOENICKE, A., LÖFFLER, B., KUGLER, J., STUTTMANN, H. and GROTE, B. (1982) Plasma concentration and the E.E.G. after various regimens of etomidate. *British Journal of Anaesthesia*, **54**, 393–400
12. SCHÜTTLER, J., SCHWILDEN, H. and STOECKEL, H. (1985) Infusion strategies to investigate the pharmacokinetics and pharmacodynamics of hypnotic drugs: etomidate as an example. *European Journal of Anaesthesiology*, **2**, 133–142
13. SCHWILDEN, H., SCHÜTTLER, J. and STOECKEL, H. (1985) Quantitation of the EEG and pharmacodynamic modelling of hypnotic drugs: etomidate as an example. *European Journal of Anaesthesiology*, **2**, 121–131
14. SCHÜTTLER, J., STANSKI, D. R., WHITE, P. F., TREVOR, A. J. and HORAI, Y. (1987) Pharmacodynamic modelling of the EEG effects of ketamine and its enantiomers in man. *Journal of Pharmacokinetics and Biopharmaceutics*, (in press)
15. SCHWILDEN, H., SCHÜTTLER, J. and STOECKEL, H. (1987)) Closed-loop feedback control of methohexital anesthesia by quantitative EEG analysis in man. *Anesthesiology* (in press)
16. HUDSON, R. J., STANSKI, D. R., SAIDMAN, L. J. and MEATHE, E. (1983) A model for studying depth of anesthesia and acute tolerance to thiopental. *Anesthesiology*, **59**, 301–308
17. SCHWILDEN, H., STOECKEL, H., SCHÜTTLER, J. and LAUVEN, P. M. (1986) Pharmacological models and their use in clinical anaesthesia. *European Journal of Anaesthesiology*, **3**, 175–208
18. MORI, K. (1973) Excitation and depression of CNS electrical activities induced by general anaesthetics. In *Proceedings of the 5th World Congress of Anaesthesiology*, edited by M. Miyazaki, K. Iwatsaki and M. Fujita, pp. 40–53. Amsterdam: Excerpta Medica
19. SCHWILDEN, H. and STOECKEL, H. (1987) Quantitative EEG analysis with isoflurane in nitrous oxide at 1.3 and 1.5 MAC. *British Journal of Anaesthesia*, (in press)
20. SCHWILDEN, H. and STOECKEL, H. (1986) Quantitating the EEG effect of volatile anaesthetics. *European Journal of Anaesthesiology*, (Abstract) **3**, 40–41
21. STOECKEL, H. and SCHWILDEN, H. (1984) Quantitative EEG analysis and monitoring depth of anaesthesia. In *Proceedings of the 8th World Congress of Anaesthesiologists*, edited by Q. J. Gomez, L. M. Egay and M. F. de la Cruz-Odi, pp. 151–158. Amsterdam: Excerpta Medica

Chapter 8

The cerebral function analysing monitor: principles and potential use

M. Frank and P. F. Prior

The cerebral function analysing monitor (CFAM*) was developed by Maynard[1,2] as a second generation system for monitoring EEG and evoked potentials. It grew from the cerebral function monitor (CFM†)[3], which had proved a robust EEG monitor in clinical practice but lacked the sophistication required in some, notably anaesthetic, applications. The principles of the methods used for acquisition, processing and display of data are based on considerable research into the fundamental characteristics of the electrical activity of the brain and considerable experience of clinical monitoring. This has led to a system which differs from most others available in several important respects which may be summarized as follows:

- EEG amplitude and frequency content are analysed and displayed separately.
- Measurements can be made from the chart and a digital output is also provided via an RS232C interface.
- A special filter counteracts the inherent tendency of the slower waves of the EEG to be of higher voltage than the faster ones and so distort the analysis.
- Frequency information is expressed as a percentage of the total in each of the conventional EEG frequency bands. This means that even very low amplitude signals may be assessed accurately from the display when absolute values would be virtually invisible.
- The low amplitude traces are clearly displayed and periods of suppression falling below chosen thresholds indicated. Variability of the signal is also evident. These features ensure that burst suppression pattern and brief high voltage peaks (for example during arousal or seizure discharges) can be promptly recognized.
- Immediate display of the unprocessed EEG is available.
- The state of the electrode contact resistance, presence of line frequency interference, occurrence of scalp muscle potentials and artefacts affecting the signal pathway, are indicated.
- Evoked potentials to sensory stimuli may be averaged and displayed on the same chart as the EEG and may be monitored automatically at chosen intervals.

Principles of the method

The initial CFAM signal processing[1,2,4,5] is similar to that of the original CFM from which it was developed. Essentially, the EEG is weighted by a prewhitening filter based on investigation of the frequency analysis of the normal EEG[6], which

*, † see p. 71

gives something nearer to equal weight to all frequencies. The signal is then subjected to logarithmic amplitude compression and envelope detection retaining the DC component. The amplitude distribution is then measured. To enhance trends, a backward weighted mean is given for the mean and for the 90th and 10th centile values. The maxima and minima outside those centile values are individually superimposed every 2 seconds to highlight brief peaks or brief suppressions. Burst suppression activity is processed so that total suppressions or silent periods give a near zero microvolt output and each burst a deflection proportional to its peak-to-peak amplitude. Frequency analysis derived from a baseline crossing technique is written out as the percentage of the total falling in each frequency band. This use of a percentage, or relative frequency measure, makes possible analysis and display of the frequency content of very low voltage activity, including less than $1\,\mu V$; absolute frequency values may be calculated by reference to the mean amplitude. Such a display also gives a good indication of the variability of each parameter. The possibility of alternating between two recording sites also allows useful visual comparisons, for example between the two hemispheres in a patient during carotid surgery.

Sensory evoked potential monitoring is also possible with sequential display alternating with or replacing the EEG analysis. For pure evoked potential monitoring, there may be advantages in using other forms of display such as those resembling a compressed spectral array[7, 8], which would conveniently highlight the type of changes with volatile agents discussed by Professor Jones in Chapter 12. It has to be noted that the ability of evoked potentials, however displayed, to depict the moment of arousal or wakening is much less certain. Probably the appearance of later cortical components would give the only means of predicting that this might be imminent. That would require longer sweep times for averaging. There is, as yet, no published quantitative study of evoked potentials at different depths of anaesthesia using the CFAM, and this facility will not be referred to further.

Changes during anaesthesia

Both the inter- and intra-individual variability in the EEG frequency distribution seen in an awake patient changes towards a more uniform pattern when anaesthesia is induced, irrespective of the anaesthetic agent used[9]. During 'light' levels of anaesthesia, fast activity (beta) predominates in the EEG signal (*Figure 8.1*). With the administration of increasing doses of anaesthetic agent there is a shift towards lower frequencies until burst suppression appears, which consists of bursts of

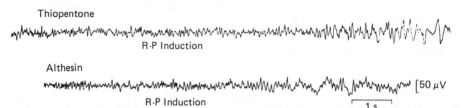

Thiopentone

R-P Induction

Althesin

R-P Induction

$[50\,\mu V$

1 s

Figure 8.1 Conventional EEG recordings from two patients during anaesthetic induction with two different intravenous anaesthetic agents. Time runs from left to right, each sample lasting approximately 10 s. Recordings are from right parietal [R-P] scalp electrodes. Note how the faster waves seen initially are replaced by slower and larger waves as anaesthesia is induced. The two agents produce remarkably similar EEG changes. Recordings continue in *Figure 8.2*. (Reproduced by kind permission of D. F. Scott and S. Virden[9])

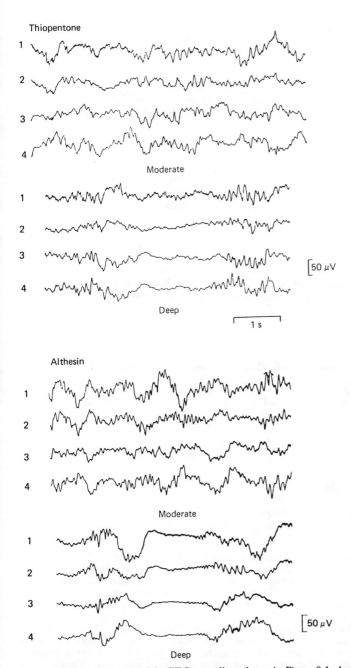

Figure 8.2 A continuation of the EEG recordings shown in *Figure 8.1*, showing changes with increasing depth of anaesthesia. Each of the four samples of tracing is similarly recorded, from frontal to occipital regions, channels 1 to 4. During 'moderate' anaesthesia a mixture of frequencies including high voltage slow waves is present. With 'deep' anaesthesia, a burst suppression pattern is present. Note how the amplitude fluctuates between periods of high (the bursts), and very low (suppressions) amplitude. There is considerable similarity in the EEG effects of the two agents. (Reproduced by kind permission of D. F. Scott and S. Virden[9])

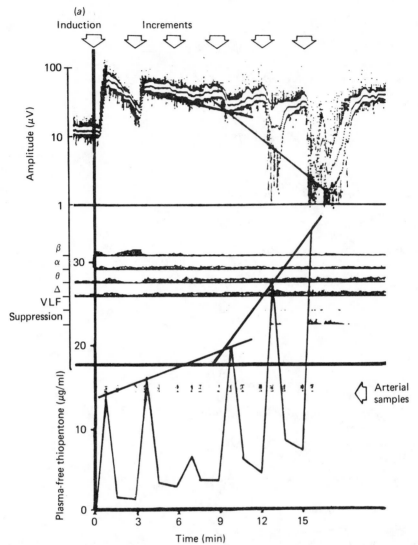

Figure 8.3 CFAM traces of patients who received intravenous bolus injections of (*a*) thiopentone, and (*b*) ICI 35 868. Note the marked similarity in the traces obtained with the two drugs, and also the 'induction peak' in the amplitude signal, followed by a second smaller similar peak after the second bolus injection. Thereafter, the amplitude drops further after each successive injection until the pattern of burst suppression becomes evident, characterized by a broad trace which reflects the wide fluctuations of cerebral energy output, and resting close to the baseline, corresponding to the suppressions. The frequency distribution shows a high percentage of beta activity initially (except for a brief attenuation during the peak of induction), and during the 'recovery' period after each injection decreasing at each successive interval as drug levels accumulate. Percentage of delta follows the opposite trend, increasing successively after each injection. Burst suppression activity is represented by a predominance of the lower frequencies including 'VLF' and 'Suppression'. Circulating levels of the anaesthetic are shown to have a negative relationship with the amplitude signal after the third injection (the third thiopentone peak was missed due to late sampling). Changes in the frequency distribution are consistent, including the first two bolus intervals in 'light' anaesthesia. (Reproduced with the permission of the authors[11,12] and the Editors of the *British Journal of Anaesthesia* and of the *European Journal of Anaesthesiology*)

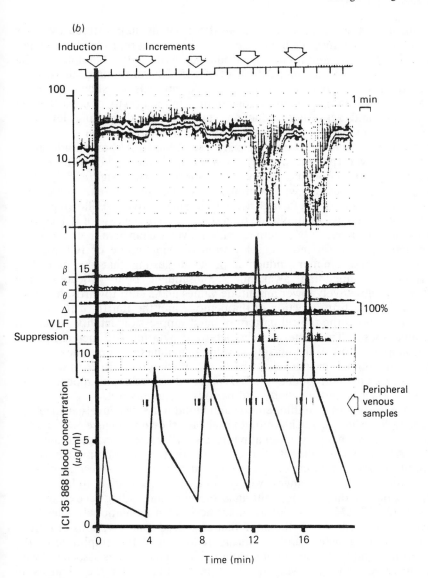

Figure 8.3 continued

electrical activity interspersed with periods of near or total electrical silence (*Figure 8.2*). With a further increase in anaesthetic depth, the bursts of activity become progressively less frequent and finally disappear leaving an isoelectric trace.

A preliminary study during Althesin (alphaxalone–alphadalone) anaesthesia in the baboon, compared a prototype CFAM with a CFM and with conventional EEG displayed in a compressed form and assessed by computer for incidence of burst suppression activity. An analysis of variance showed significant differences between the measurements at six different depths of anaesthesia. These could be well characterized by the CFAM[10].

Single drug studies using intravenous anaesthetic agents administered by bolus doses[11-13] or by steady infusion[14] have shown consistent and reproducible changes in the CFAM (or CFM) amplitude and frequency write-outs. Examples of the CFAM signal obtained when thiopentone or ICI 35 868 were administered on a weight-related basis at a specified rate at 4-minute intervals are shown in *Figure 8.3*. The rapid changes in the signal are consistent with the brevity of clinical effect of these agents, and represent induction, followed by deepening levels of anaesthesia alternating with rapid recovery after each bolus injection.

Anaesthetic induction is followed by a sharp rise of the CFAM amplitude signal from its resting level (patient awake) to a peak, coincidental with loss of consciousness, 20–30 s after the intravenous injection (*see Figure 8.3*). This 'induction peak' is associated with a transient attenuation of beta percentage activity and an increase of theta and delta frequency activity. Following these changes, there is a decrease in amplitude (at a slower rate in the case of ICI 35 868), and a considerable increase of beta activity with a reverse change in theta and delta percentage activity. The second bolus injection of thiopentone or ICI 35 868 is followed by a second, smaller 'induction peak' suggesting that the preceding changes represent impending awakening. Subsequent bolus injections are associated with progressively lower amplitude values and a shift towards the lower frequencies. After the fifth injection of thiopentone and the fourth of ICI 35 868, the CFAM signal shows the typical pattern of burst suppression activity associated with deep anaesthesia. The pattern is characterized by a marked increase in the width of the amplitude trace, the maximum value signalling the amplitude of bursts of activity and the minimum, periods of EEG suppression near $0\,\mu V$. In addition, this is demonstrated in the frequency analysis part of the trace by the appearance of increasing very low frequency activity and periods of suppression.

Plasma concentration of free thiopentone and blood ICI 35 868 levels at specified blood sampling times during each 4-minute cycle are shown in *Figure 8.3*, and the relationship between changing circulating levels of anaesthetic agent and the changing CFAM signal is evident. Closer correlations were obtained between CFAM amplitude and circulating drug levels with increasing anaesthesia, while the beta and delta frequency changes were found to be sensitive indicators of anaesthetic depth including during light anaesthesia or impending recovery[11-13].

Changes in the CFAM signal during anaesthesia with inhalational anaesthetic agents have been described[15, 16]. Subanaesthetic inspired concentrations of nitrous oxide resulted in a consistent and significant reduction of the amplitude of the CFAM recording, and the cessation of nitrous oxide inhalation was associated with a marked increase and overswing of the CFAM amplitude; the changes in percentage frequency activity were variable. Anaesthesia with halothane was associated with an increase in amplitude at 1 MAC (MAC = minimal alveolar concentration at which 50% subjects react to a specified stimulus), and a decrease at 2 MAC, while the frequency distribution showed a progressive decrease in beta activity with an increase in delta activity with increasing concentrations of halothane. This pattern follows the same trend as that seen with the intravenous drugs.

In a clinical study (P. Dodd, M. Frank and D. E. Maynard, unpublished data), cerebral electrical activity was monitored with the CFAM in a group of patients who underwent extracorporeal shock wave lithotripsy under light general anaesthesia. This provided suitable conditions to observe the effect on the CFAM signal of the shock wave, which is a uniform stimulus continually triggered by the R wave of the ECG. The stimulus of the shock wave has both auditory and painful somatosensory components. The patients were unpremedicated, they received a midazolam–thiopentone intravenous induction, anaesthesia was maintained solely with nitrous oxide (in oxygen) and enflurane, and the patients were paralysed and their lungs ventilated ($PE'CO_2$: 3.2–3.5 kPa). Examples of the CFAM trace at the commencement of the shock wave stimulus are shown in *Figure 8.4*. The first

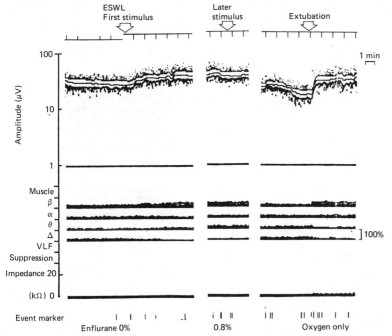

Figure 8.4 Portions of a CFAM trace obtained from a patient who was anaesthetized for extracorporeal shock wave lithotripsy showing the characteristic 'alerting' response, consisting of a change in amplitude and an increase in beta activity, at the commencement of treatment and during extubation at the conclusion of the procedure. These changes were absent at a subsequent application of the shock wave stimulus when more anaesthetic had been administered

application of the stimulus resulted in an increase of the amplitude and of the percentage beta activity and an attenuation of delta activity. This CFAM pattern has been observed on other occasions when a stimulus of marked intensity is applied to a patient who has received low doses of anaesthetic agents, and who may show other signs (e.g. cardiovascular) of light anaesthesia. A subsequent application of the shock wave stimulus did not visibly alter either the amplitude or the frequency signals. This lack of response was associated with an increased inspired concentration of enflurane and presumed corresponding changes in anaesthetic depth. On completing the extracorporeal shock wave lithotripsy treatment and cessation of the anaesthetic, tracheal extubation caused a marked increase in the CFAM amplitude and beta activity signals, similar to the trend described when the stimulus was first applied under light anaesthesia.

A logical extension of the microprocessor-based system of the CFAM is the delineation of profiles of inadequate anaesthesia which could be used to generate warnings. Recording protocols can be preset for particular anaesthetic procedures or research projects. Analysis could characterize normative EEG and evoked potential profiles for increasing depths of individual anaesthetics. It was envisaged that this would permit informed control of a chosen agent using feedback to the anaesthetist rather than automatic delivery of anaesthetic in the way that was investigated in the 1950s. For detection of inadequate anaesthesia, one would need to define clusters of significant variables including EEG, muscle potentials and cortical auditory evoked potentials[17]. This is what the experienced electro-encephalographer routinely does by eye; there is a considerable potential for

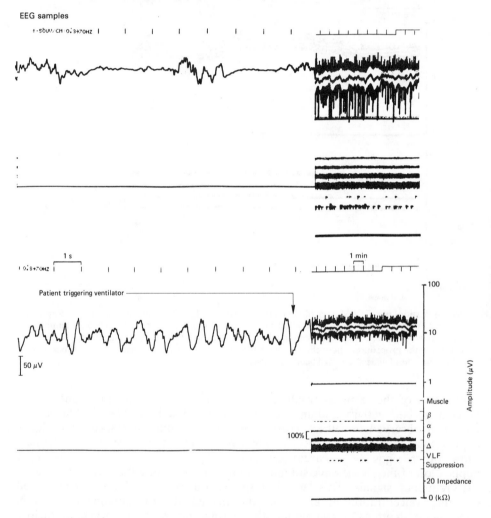

Figure 8.5 CFAM trace including two unprocessed EEG samples from a woman in posthypoxic coma, who had been given intravenous thiopentone. Two different patterns alternated; above, burst suppression activity and below, mixed slow wave activity. Note the output from the suppression index during the period of burst suppression, also a widely fluctuating amplitude from 1 to 30 µV peak to peak, which is confirmed by the corresponding EEG sample. The lower trace has a higher and narrower amplitude range; the disappearance of suppressions is confirmed in the corresponding EEG sample

defining and quantifying this expertise and making it available as preprogrammed 'learned' memory. Such a multivariate, or pattern recognition, approach would permit automatic detection of momentary changes or alterations in variability, occurring as responses to surgical or auditory stimuli.

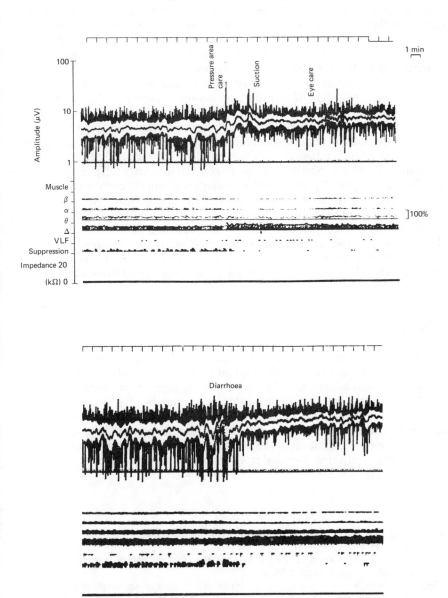

Figure 8.6 The effect of external and presumed internal stimuli on the CFAM trace of the patient described in *Figure 8.5*. The upper trace shows the abolition of burst suppression pattern at the time of 'care of pressure areas' followed by tracheal suction. The lower trace obtained a few hours later shows a similar change; it coincided with an attack of diarrhoea which would presumably have been accompanied by colicky abdominal pains

Use in the intensive care unit

Clinical applications of the CFAM include situations in which it is important to monitor altered patterns of cerebral activity which occur in association with unconscious states. These include pharmacologically induced cerebral depression, as in controlled sedation in the intensive care unit, or drug overdose, and cerebral dysfunction whether transient or long term resulting from hypoxia and other metabolic encephalopathies, hypotension, or trauma. Increased cerebral activity in status epilepticus and the effectiveness of the appropriate anticonvulsant therapy may be monitored by the CFAM's continuous visual display.

An example of the clinical use in the intensive care unit of the CFAM to monitor cerebral activity and the effect of noxious stimulation, is shown in *Figures 8.5* and *8.6*. These show portions of a continuous CFAM trace obtained from a patient over a period of 4 weeks following cardiac arrest and hypoxic brain damage, manifested by a prolonged period of coma and frequent grand mal seizures. The patient received an intravenous infusion of thiopentone. Throughout the period of monitoring, the CFAM tracing alternated between two distinctly different patterns. These are shown in *Figure 8.5* which include samples of unprocessed EEG in each state: bursts suppression pattern and continuous mixed slow wave activity. Sometimes it was evident that the changes of pattern were related to changes in the rate of administration of thiopentone, but on most occasions it was coincident with external or presumed internal stimulation (*Figure 8.6*). These changes of cerebral activity, easily identifiable in the CFAM signal, can be used as a prognostic sign. Since this recording, the patient has regained consciousness and carries out simple conversations and tasks.

Conclusion

The CFAM is a comprehensive neurophysiological monitoring system. It allows the possibility of defining visually, as well as quantitatively, all depths of anaesthesia, controlled sedation and coma, as well as indicating the signs of imminent arousal or wakening. Its great advantage is that, within the compass of a single box, it is possible to generate digital data, to make a quick check of the raw EEG, or average an evoked potential. The relative simplicity of the display allows, after only minimal practice, easy recognition of the warning signs of lightening anaesthesia by anaesthetists; and the patterns obtained from patients in the intensive care unit may give some prognostic indication.

References

1. MAYNARD, D. E. (1977) The cerebral function analyser monitor (CFAM). *Electroencephalography and Clinical Neurophysiology,* **43,** 479P
2. MAYNARD, D. E. (1979) Development of the CFM: the cerebral function analysing monitor [CFAM]. *Annales de l'Anesthésiologie Française,* **20,** 253–255
3. MAYNARD, D. E., PRIOR, P. F. and SCOTT, D. F. (1969) Device for continuous monitoring of cerebral activity in resuscitated patients. *British Medical Journal,* **4,** 545–546
4. MAYNARD, D. E. and JENKINSON, J. L. (1984) The cerebral function analysing monitor. Initial clinical experience, application and further development. *Anaesthesia,* **39,** 678–690
5. PRIOR, P. F. and MAYNARD, D. E. (1986) *Monitoring Cerebral Function,* 2nd edn. Amsterdam: Elsevier

6. MAYNARD, D. E. (1969) A note on the nature of the non-rhythmic components of the electroencephalogram. *Activitas Nervosa Superior,* **11,** 238–241

7. PFURTSCHELLER, G. (1986) Monitoring of spontaneous and evoked brain activity. In *Abstracts 1, VIIth European Congress of Anaesthesiology,* edited by H. Bergman, H. Kramar and K. Steinbereithner, *Beitrage zur Anesthesiologie und Intensivmedizin,* **16,** 268–269

8. BERTRAND, O., GARCIA-LARREA, L., PERNIER, F., MAUGUIÈRE, F. and ARTRU, F. (1987) Brain-stem monitoring I. A system for high-rate sequential BAEP recording and feature extraction. *Electroencephalography and Clinical Neurophysiology* (in press)

9. SCOTT, D. F. and VIRDEN, S. (1972) Comparison of the effect of althesin with other induction agents on electroencephalographic patterns. *Postgraduate Medical Journal,* **48** (Suppl. 2), 93–96

10. PRIOR, P. F., MAYNARD, D. E. and BRIERLEY, J. B. (1978) EEG monitoring for the control of anaesthesia produced by the infusion of althesin in primates. *British Journal of Anaesthesia,* **50,** 993–1001

11. FRANK, M., MAYNARD, D. E., TSANACLIS, L. M., MAJOR, E. and COUTINHO, P. (1984) Changes in cerebral electrical activity measured by the cerebral function analysing monitor following bolus injections of thiopentone. *British Journal of Anaesthesia,* **56,** 1075–1081

12. YATE, P. M., MAYNARD, D. E., MAJOR, E., FRANK, M., VERNIQUET, A. J. W., ADAMS, H. K. and DOUGLAS, E. J. (1986) Anaesthesia with ICI 35 868 monitored by the cerebral function analysing monitor (CFAM) *European Journal of Anaesthesiology,* **3,** 159–166

13. FRANK, M., SAVEGE, T. M., LEIGH, M., GREENWOOD, J. and HOLLY, J. M. P. (1982) Comparison of the cerebral function monitor and plasma concentrations of thiopentone and alphaxalone during total i.v. anaesthesia with repeated bolus doses of thiopentone and althesin. *British Journal of Anaesthesia,* **54,** 609–616

14. MAJOR, E., VERNIQUET, A. J. W., YATE, P. M. and WADDELL, T. K. (1982) Disoprofol and fentanyl for total intravenous anaesthesia. *Anaesthesia,* **37,** 541–547

15. WILLIAMS, D. J. M., MORGAN, R. J. M., SEBEL, P. S. and MAYNARD, D. E. (1984) The effect of nitrous oxide on cerebral activity. *Anaesthesia,* **39,** 422–425

16. WARK, K. J., SEBEL, P. S., VERGHESE, C., MAYNARD, D. E. and EVANS, S. J. W. (1986) The effect of halothane on cerebral electrical activity. An assessment using the cerebral function analysing monitor (CFAM). *Anaesthesia,* **41,** 390–394

17. JONES, J. G. and KONIECZKO, K. (1986) Hearing and memory in anaesthetised patients. *British Medical Journal,* **292,** 1291–1293

* Registered Trade Mark, RDM Consultants Ltd, Unit 7, Lady Bee Marina, Southwick, Sussex BN4 4EG, UK. *UK patents* applied for. Manufactured under licence by Health Care Developments Ltd, 16 Leydon Road, Herts SG1 2BP, UK

† *UK patent* Nos. 1247491 and 1247492. *USA patent* 369947 (RE 28214). Manufactured by Lectromed Ltd, Rue Fondon, St Peter, Jersey, CI, UK.

Chapter 9

The use of the EEG to predict patient movement during anaesthesia

R. C. Dutton, W. D. Smith and N. Ty Smith

Can the EEG help to ensure that patients will not remember being aware during general anaesthesia? This question was pursued initially by the development of an EEG computer processing method which based the interpretation of data upon prediction of patient movement during general anaesthesia. The EEG system was then used in preliminary studies which correlated the EEG with recall and recognition testing: this report is a review of the work involved and which is continuing.

Our primary interest is to use the EEG to predict memory of intra-operative awareness, but awareness is a difficult end-point upon which to base an EEG system: such a system would have required a considerable number of cases of awareness. Therefore a start was made with the end-point of patient movement in response to surgical stimulation or verbal commands to avoid any possibility of unpleasant awareness. This end-point has proved to be a most reliable indicator of anaesthetic depth during numerous studies of minimum alveolar concentration[1,2]. The movement end-point is important from the standpoint of awareness, since the unparalysed patients who do not move during surgery very rarely have any memory of awareness during surgery. This means an EEG system which predicts patient movement might be used to titrate administration of anaesthetic agents and to help ensure amnesia during general anaesthesia. This EEG system would be especially useful while light general anaesthesia is maintained in paralysed patients. In a manner analogous to studies of minimum alveolar concentration, in which the concentration of anaesthetic agent is used to plot dose–response curves to describe the probability that patients will move, the EEG was used to plot curves to predict patient movement. The first step was the development of a method to express the EEG in the form of a single-number score. The EEG was analysed by parametric analysis[3] to obtain 13 parameters for describing the EEG power frequency spectrum. A computer analysis technique, called discriminant analysis, was then used to determine the best method to use the 13 parameters for scoring the EEG in order to predict patient movement. These scores were then used to generate probability of patient-movement curves, similar to quantal response curves[4]. These curves could be used to convert any EEG score into a probability of patient movement. This gave three ways of describing the EEG in terms of: 13 parameters of the power frequency spectrum, a single-number score, and a probability of patient movement. The probability of movement curves could also be used to compare the EEG effects of anaesthetic agents and to compare the sensitivity of the EEG scoring method used with the sensitivity of other methods.

Patient selection and anaesthetic techniques

The EEG was monitored in 150 healthy women, aged between 18 and 42 years, who were to have elective laparoscopy as outpatients. The patients did not receive any premedication. Anaesthesia was induced with thiopentone 4 mg/kg and maintained with either isoflurane in 70% nitrous oxide, isoflurane–fentanyl 4 µg/kg (without nitrous oxide), or fentanyl 4 µg/kg and 70% nitrous oxide. (If patients moved, additional thiopentone and/or isoflurane were administered.) The only muscle relaxants administered were tubocurarine 3 mg to reduce fasciculation and suxamethonium 1.5 mg/kg for tracheal intubation. Patients' lungs were ventilated at a rate of 9 per min and with a tidal volume of 8–10 ml/kg. End-tidal CO_2 was not measured. The concentration of inspired isoflurane was read from a calibrated isoflurane vaporizer and fresh gas flow was 5 ℓ/min.

EEG computer processing method

One bipolar EEG channel was recorded from silver/silver chloride electrodes pasted to the forehead (FP1 area) and left ear. The EEG signal was amplified, filtered (2–30 Hz), and digitized for analysis on an Apple II+ computer. A

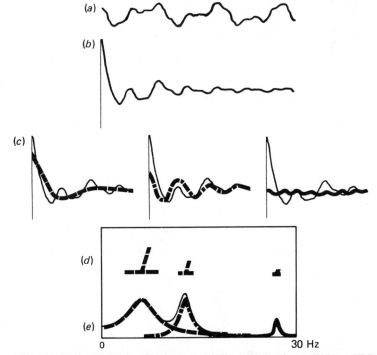

Figure 9.1 Pictorial representation of parametric analysis. An epoch of raw EEG (*a*) is processed to find its autocorrelation function (*b*) which contains information about the EEG power frequency spectrum. The autocorrelation curve is then resolved into components (*c*), each of which gives the spectral component parameters (centre frequency, half-width, and power) of a peak in the spectrum. The spectral component parameters can be displayed directly (*d*) or can be used to plot a continuous power spectrum curve (*e*)

parametric analysis method (*Figure 9.1*) was used to determine a data record consisting of 13 parameters of the power frequency spectrum for each 15-second epoch of EEG. The parameters were the root mean square voltage and the centre frequency, half-bandwidth, and relative power for each of up to four peaks of spectral components in the power spectrum. Each data record was displayed on line in the operating room (*Figure 9.2*), and the data records were also stored on a small floppy disk for later analysis.

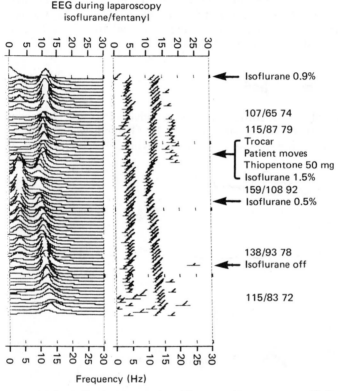

Figure 9.2 Recording from one patient. The spectral parameters are displayed in the operating room (right column). Each data record, displayed horizontally in the figure, is for a 15-second epoch, with time advancing downward. The corresponding power spectra are included for comparison (left column)

EEG scoring method

The following section describes the methodology used to develop the EEG score. The end result is that the 13 parameters of the EEG spectrum can be recombined into a single-number score between 0 and 100.

A 60-second period (i.e. four epochs) was selected just before the insertion of the trocar, since it is desirable to predict patient movement. The EEG data were called 'move/trocar' or 'no move/trocar' which depended on the patient's response to trocar insertion. The concentration of inspired isoflurane could be reduced considerably before any additional movement was likely to occur following trocar insertion. The later portion of the laparoscopy was called 'closing'; a 60-second period before any movement or response or, if there was no movement or response, a 60-second period of the lightest appearing EEG was also selected: these data were called 'move/closing' or 'no move/closing'. Thus, the EEG data consist of 12 groups (six pairs) of records: the pair 'move/trocar' and 'no move/trocar' and the pair 'move/closing' and 'no move/closing' for each of the three anaesthetic techniques. *Figure 9.3* shows some of the data from one of the pairs of groups.

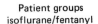

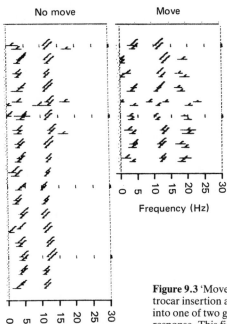

Figure 9.3 'Move' and 'no move' groups. The data records just before trocar insertion are extracted from each patient's recording and placed into one of two groups: 'move' or 'no move', according to the patient's response. This figure shows two data records for each of 18 'no move' and nine 'move' patients

Discriminant analysis is a computer method for determining the best way to use the variables of data records to separate the records into known groups[5]. The 13 parameters for each EEG record are first reduced to six variables to prepare for discriminant analysis. Some parameters were found to be useful variables as they

$$\text{Score} = -42A_\delta + 71H_\alpha + 25A_{\beta1+2} + 34A_{\beta2}$$
$$-131\,\text{PK} + 12\,\text{SP} + 43$$

Figure 9.4 Discriminant function. This discriminant function uses six variables with their coefficients and a constant. The variables are: A = relative power of peaks in 0–7.5 Hz range, H = height of peak in 7.5–13.5 Hz range, $A_{\beta1+2}$ = relative power in peaks > 13.5 Hz, $A_{\beta2}$ = relative power in peaks > 22.5 Hz, PK = a measure of the sharpness of the spectral peaks, and SP = a measure of the uniformity of power distribution among peaks. This discriminant function is used to score data records on a scale from 0 to 100

were, but others were found to be most useful when combined to form new variables. A discriminant analysis program was then given the six variables for each record of 'move' and 'no move' groups and instructed to determine the discriminant function, in terms of the coefficients which maximized the separation of the groups (*Figure 9.4*). The resulting discriminant function then became the method for scoring the EEG data records.

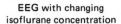

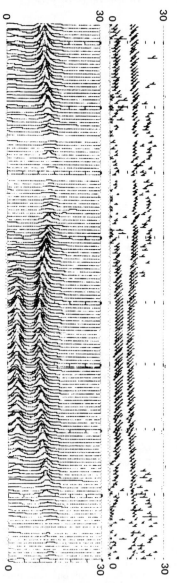

Figure 9.5 EEG with changing isoflurane. This is the recording from one patient receiving isoflurane–fentanyl anaesthesia. Each data record is for a 15-second epoch, with time advancing downward. The inspired isoflurane concentration was equilibrated at 0.9% and then, changing 0.25%/min, decreased to 0.1%, increased to 1.9%, and returned to 0.1%

A common scoring system for EEG data from the three anaesthetic techniques was sought. There were considerable shifts, similar to those previously reported[6], in the EEG spectra of patients from a broad range of isoflurane concentrations (*Figure 9.5*). The authors' rather arbitrary initial approach, then, was to select four pairs of 'move' and 'no move' data that seemed to correspond to different states along the shifting spectrum: the 'move' and 'no move'/trocar/isoflurane–nitrous oxide spectra showed predominantly low frequencies; the 'move' and 'no move'/trocar/isoflurane–fentanyl spectra included some higher frequency activity; the 'move' and 'no move'/closing/isoflurane–fentanyl spectra even higher frequencies; and the 'move' and 'no move'/closing/fentanyl–nitrous oxide spectra showed predominantly high frequencies. Instead of instructing discriminant analysis to separate groups that were not a 'move'/'no move' pair, but were adjacent to each other, such as the 'move'/trocar/isoflurane–nitrous oxide and the 'no move'/trocar/isoflurane–fentanyl groups, it was decided to combine them into one group. In this way, the original eight groups were reduced to five groups – two of the original groups (at the upper and lower ends of the spectral shifting), and three combined groups. Discriminant analysis was then applied to the five groups.

The discriminant function coefficients were scaled so that an EEG of pure delta activity had a score of 0, and a power frequency spectrum of equal activity across the spectrum had a score of 80; nearly all the EEG data records could be expressed as a number from 0 to 100 (*see Figure 9.4*). An occasional data record would be greater than 100 or less than 0, and burst suppression was arbitrarily assigned a value of 0.

Probability-of-move curves

Using the EEG scores, a probability-of-move curve was generated for trocar/isoflurane–fentanyl data from nine patients who moved and 42 patients who did not move. A similar curve was plotted for closing/isoflurane–fentanyl data from

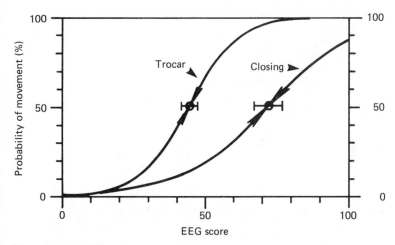

Figure 9.6 Probability of movement for trocar and closing with isoflurane–fentanyl. Each curve is based on EEG scores from 51 patients. Confidence limits (one standard deviation of the estimate) are shown at the point of 50% probability of movement, for the score and for the slope

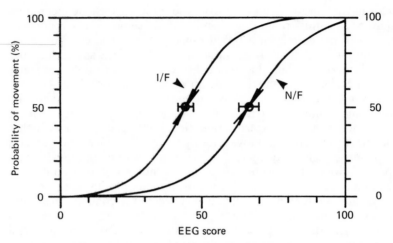

Figure 9.7 Probability of movement for trocar for isoflurane–fentanyl (I/F) and fentanyl–nitrous oxide (N/F). The confidence limits are the same as in *Figure 9.6*

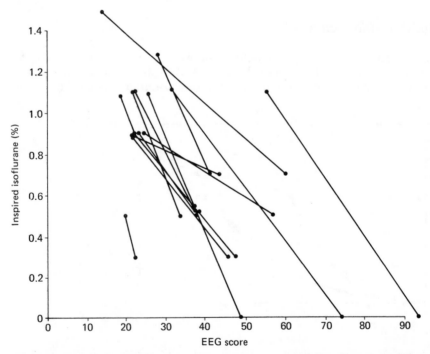

Figure 9.8 EEG score and isoflurane concentration. The change in EEG score with change in inspired isoflurane concentration, is shown for each of 14 patients receiving isoflurane–fentanyl 4 µg/kg anaesthesia

equal numbers of patients (*Figure 9.6*). Probability-of-move curves were also generated for other anaesthetic techniques (*Figure 9.7*).

The next step was to compare the discriminant function scoring method with other methods of scoring the EEG. The most sensitive scoring method would be the method where the smallest change in isoflurane concentration produced a given change in probability of movement predicted by the EEG score. To calculate this change in isoflurane concentration, the change in EEG score necessary for a change in probability of movement from 50% to 20% was determined, and then the change in inspired isoflurane concentration necessary to produce this change in EEG score was determined. For example, this change in probability of movement, as shown in *Figure 9.6*, requires a change in EEG score from 44 to 32. *Figure 9.8* shows the changes in EEG scores when the inspired isoflurane concentration is changed during isoflurane–fentanyl anaesthesia. Using the median slope in *Figure 9.8*, a change of score of 44 to 32 requires a change in inspired isoflurane of 0.25%. Thus, it requires a change in inspired isoflurane of 0.25% to reduce the probability of move from 50% to 20% during trocar insertion.

Two other commonly used EEG scoring methods, the median or 50% power frequency (F_{50}) and the 90% power frequency (F_{90}), can also be calculated from our parametric analysis. For the F_{50} and F_{90} scoring methods, the change in inspired isoflurane for change in probability of movement from 50% to 20% was calculated by going through similar processes of generating probability-of-move curves for F_{50} and F_{90}, and curves showing changes in F_{50} and F_{90} when the inspired concentration of isoflurane was changed. These results are given in *Table 9.1*, and show that the discriminant function is the most sensitive of the three scoring methods for isoflurane–fentanyl anaesthesia, at the anaesthetic depth where 20–50% of patients would be predicted to move at the moment of trocar insertion. The discriminant function scoring method was also found to be the most sensitive during lighter anaesthesia where 20–50% of patients would be predicted to move during the closing phase. During isoflurane–nitrous oxide, for both trocar and closing, the discriminant function scoring method was the most sensitive of the three methods.

Table 9.1 Change in inspired isoflurane concentration for change in probability of movement from 50% to 20%

	Inspired isoflurane concn (%)
Discriminant function	0.25
F_{50}	0.32
F_{90}	0.52

Patient responsiveness to verbal stimuli

Patients were, in addition, observed for responsiveness when their names were called and they were asked to squeeze their hands. Of 27 patients who moved at the time of trocar insertion, 26 patients moved in response to surgical stimulation, and one patient, who did not move in response to surgical stimulation, did open her eyes when her name was called. Of 27 patients who moved during the closing phase, 18 patients moved in response to surgical stimulation, and nine patients moved when their names were called, even though they had not been moving in response to surgical stimulation. Three of these nine patients also squeezed their hands when requested to do so. The patients who responded to their names, but not surgical stimulation, were receiving either isoflurane–fentanyl or fentanyl–nitrous oxide anaesthesia.

It is interesting to wonder whether the patients who moved with surgical stimulation would have lower EEG scores than patients who responded to their names. *Table 9.2* shows median scores and ranges for these two groups of patients who received the same anaesthetic during the closing phase. There was no significant difference between groups for either anaesthetic technique.

Table 9.2 EEG scores during closing phase median, range, and number of patients

Anaesthetic	Moves with surgery			Responds to name		
	Median EEG score	Range	No. of patients	Median EEG score	Range	No. of patients
Isoflurane–fentanyl	65	47–50	4	67	48–95	5
Fentanyl–nitrous oxide	83	60–106	5	87	80–108	4

Recall and recognition

In a preliminary study with 36 female patients who had one of the three anaesthetic techniques, a simple multiple-choice recognition test was used to look for correlation between the EEG and any evidence of memory during anaesthesia. The patient's name was called during anaesthesia, and she was asked to listen to, and remember, a tape-recorded sound. The tape-recorded sound was presented to the patient during the later portion of the surgery while the patient was quite lightly anaesthetized. Three to six hours after surgery, patients were asked if they recalled the sound or any event during surgery. They were then given a recognition test in which they were asked to listen to five tape-recorded sounds, one of which was the sound they actually heard, and to guess which sound was played during surgery. These data are preliminary, and the recognition testing was not double blind, that is, the investigator knew which sound was played, but the results are interesting.

No patients recalled the tape-recorded sound or any events during surgery, even though many patients were so lightly anaesthetized that they moved during surgery, and some patients opened their eyes and squeezed their hands when requested to do so. One patient told a relative the correct sound during early emergence from anaesthesia, although she did not recall the sound when asked later. She did clearly recognize the sound on the recognition test, as did five other patients. All patients who said they clearly recognized the sound, also guessed the correct sound.

Two of these six patients, who may have remembered the sound, were moving in response to surgery at the time the sound was played, while the other four patients were not moving and did not respond to their names. The EEG scores of these six patients were relatively high. These EEG scores can be converted to a probability of movement using the trocar probability-of-move curve appropriate for each patient's anaesthetic technique. Expressed in this way, the median probability of movement for the six patients who may have remembered was 90% with a range of 72–95%. This indicates that the patients were lightly anaesthetized and, even though four patients were not moving, they would be very likely to move with a strong surgical stimulation such as the trocar insertion.

Discussion

This chapter describes work in progress. The discriminant function developed by the authors for scoring the EEG is a current version that best fits their relatively small database. A different discriminant function would be obtained if different variables were chosen or if the database shifted when more patient data were added. Data were used from three different anaesthetic techniques to obtain a discriminant function applicable to a wide range of data. Alternatively, a discriminant function could be developed using the data for a specific anaesthetic technique.

This discriminant function showed greater sensitivity than the median frequency or the 90% power frequency. While the authors' calculation of F_{50} and F_{90} was made from parametric analysis data, and the usual calculation of F_{50} and F_{90} is made from Fourier analysis data, there is a very close correlation between the results calculated by both methods (W. D. Smith, unpublished data).

It was always striking to witness an unparalysed patient during surgery without movement in response to surgical stimulation, yet opening her eyes and sometimes even squeezing her hand upon request. Some of these patients had elevations of blood pressure and heart rate, but many did not show any autonomic nervous system hyperactivity. The EEG score did demonstrate that these patients were very lightly anaesthetized.

The authors plan to improve their method to determine post-operative recall, recognition, or any evidence of learning. The EEG scoring method should allow better quantification of anaesthetic levels where there is no recall or recognition on memory tests, and where there might be evidence of the sort of learning described by Bennett, Davis and Giannini[7], Goldman (Chapter 16), Stolz, Couture and Edmonds[8], and Millar and Watkinson[9].

Acknowledgements

Research was supported in part by The Community Service Program of Kaiser Foundation Hospital.

Study protocol was approved by The Kaiser Permanente Medical Care Program, Northern California Regional Institutional Review Board.

References

1. EGER, E. I., SAIDMAN, L. J. and BRANDSTATER, B. (1965) Minimum alveolar anesthetic concentration: a standard of anesthetic potency. *Anesthesiology*, **26**, 756–763
2. STOELTING, R. K., LONGNECKER, D. E. and EGER, E. I. (1970) Minimum alveolar concentrations in man on awakening and methoxyflurane, halothane, ether and fluroxene anesthesia: MAC awake. *Anesthesiology*, **33**, 5–9
3. SMITH, W. D. and LAGER, D. L. (1986) Evaluation of simple algorithms for spectral parameter analysis of the electroencephalogram. *IEEE Transactions of Biomedical Engineering*, **33**, 352–358

4. WAUD, D. R. (1972) On biological assays involving quantal responses. *Journal of Pharmacology and Experimental Therapeutics,* **183**, 577–607
5. NIE, N. H., HULL, C. H., JENKINS, J. G., STEINBRENNER, K. and BENT, D. H. (1985) *SPSS: Statistical Package for the Social Sciences,* 2nd edn. New York: McGraw-Hill
6. RAMPIL, I. J. and SMITH, N. T. (1985) Comparison of EEG indices during halothane anaesthesia. *Journal of Clinical Monitoring,* **1**, 89–90
7. BENNETT, H. L., DAVIS, H. S. and GIANNINI, J. A. (1985) Non-verbal response to intraoperative conversation. *British Journal of Anaesthesia,* **57**, 174–179
8. STOLZ, S., COUTURE, L. J. and EDMONDS, H. L. JR (1985) Evidence of partial recall during general aaesthesia. *Anesthesia and Analgesia,* **65**, S154
9. MILLAR, K. and WATKINSON, N. (1983) Recognition of words presented during general anaesthesia. *Ergonomics,* **26**, 585–594

Chapter 10

The EMG, the EEG zero crossing frequency and mean integrated voltage analysis during sleep and anaesthesia

L. Herregods and G. Rolly

Assessment of unconsciousness relies mainly upon clinical signs. However, these are variable and depend on the use of particular anaesthetics, muscle relaxants and mechanical ventilation[1]. The purpose of this chapter is to demonstrate how intra-operative monitoring of cranial biopotentials was assessed in relation to unconsciousness and awareness. In the authors' department the Anaesthesia and Brain activity Monitor (ABM) of Datex is used for this purpose and was chosen because of its relative simplicity and because analysis of both EEGs and EMGs is possible. The ABM provides parallel displays of end-tidal carbon dioxide, cardiovascular variables and the neuromuscular response to train-of-four stimulation.

Materials and methods

Eight volunteers were monitored during physiological sleep and 120 patients received different anaesthetics. Informed consent was obtained from the patients and the study was approved by the Ethical Committee of the authors' hospital.

The ABM analyses the biopotentials obtained from three adhesive electrodes placed on the mid-forehead and behind the ear. A portion of the signal is high-pass

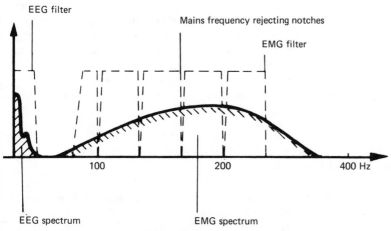

Figure 10.1 Biopotential filtration for EEG and spontaneous EMG

filtered (70–300 Hz) to obtain a spontaneous frontalis muscle EMG. Low-pass filtering (1.5–25 Hz) is used to produce the EEG (*Figure 10.1*).

Out of the raw EEG signal, a constant time period of 1 second is considered. Each time the raw EEG signal crosses the isoelectric line, an impulse is sent to the computer. The total number of these pulses, divided by the time epoch expressed in seconds, gives a number called the zero crossing frequency, expressed in hertz. The zero crossing frequency is a value for the mean frequency of the EEG signal during the considered time interval (*Figure 10.2*).

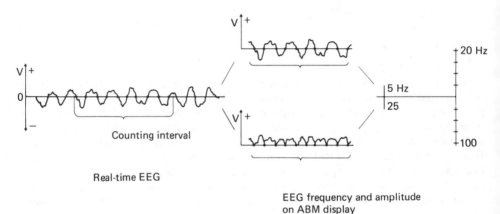

Figure 10.2 Computing of real time EEG, into zero crossing frequency and mean integrated voltage

Out of the same signal, the negative voltage part of the signal is brought to the positive side and the area under the curve is integrated. This gives an unexpressed number, the mean integrated voltage, which is a mean value of the amplitude of the EEG signal. It is a relative value between 0 and 100, which corresponds, on a non-linear scale, to between 0 and 50 μV.

The EEG signal is described by both these numbers: the 0 crossing frequency for the mean frequency and the mean integrated voltage for the mean amplitude. The electrical activity of the frontalis muscle is used to assess the spontaneous EMG. Out of the information filtered between 70 and 300 Hz, the same procedure is followed to compute the mean amplitude of this spontaneous EMG signal. This means that the integrated area under the curve is used as a mean value for the spontaneous EMG amplitude. The EMG is expressed in arbitrary units between 0 and 100 and corresponds, on a non-linear scale, to between 0 and 15 μV.

These combined monitors of EEG variables, the zero crossing frequency and mean integrated voltage provide information about the electrical activity of the brain.

Results during physiological sleep

Falling asleep, combined with a loss of consciousness, is characterized by a gradual decrease in EMG value, a less important decrease in zero crossing frequency and later an increase in mean integrated voltage. During sleep the EMG remains low. Awareness, or at least recall during sleep, as assessed by later interview, is characterized by an EMG increase to more than 60, with or without zero crossing frequency and mean integrated voltage changes. Other causes of increasing EMG are movements of the subjects and coughing (*Figure 10.3*).

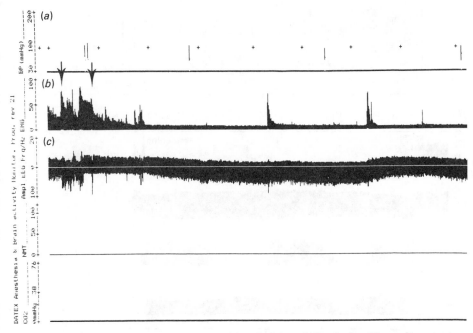

Figure 10.3 Example of a registration during physiological sleep during the first 2 hours (from top to bottom): (*a*) systolic and diastolic blood pressures (lines); (*b*) spontaneous EMG; (*c*) EEG: zero crossing frequency, above 0 line; mean integrated voltage under 0 line. At the first arrow, the subject drops off; at the second arrow, he falls asleep

No significant changes were seen either in the EEG or in the EMG recordings during the different stages of sleep. A classic hypnogram cannot be composed from the authors' recordings. It can be postulated that arousal and consciousness during or after physiological sleep is demonstrated by the EMG almost resuming its original values.

Results during anaesthetic practice

During induction, the EMG signal decreases abruptly to 10% of its conscious value. Different induction agents may have different patterns, but the loss of consciousness is always indicated by a low EMG value (between 7 and 15) (*Figure 10.4*). These changes are coincident with the loss of consciousness but are noticed before the loss of the eyelash reflex[2].

With adequate anaesthesia, and in the absence of artefacts due to interference of surgical instruments, this low amplitude persists until the end of the procedure. The EMG can be influenced by neuromuscular relaxants, which diminish the responsiveness of all skeletal muscles. However, muscles vary in their sensitivities

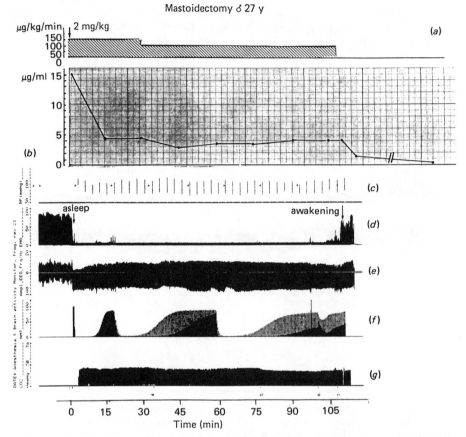

Figure 10.4 Example of a clinical anaesthesia procedure using propofol as continuous infusion (from top to bottom): (*a*) administration rate; (*b*) corresponding blood concentrations; (*c*) systolic and diastolic blood pressures (lines) and heart rate (dots); (*d*) spontaneous EMG; (*e*) EEG: zero crossing frequency, above 0 line; mean integrated voltage, under 0 line; (*f*) neuromuscular monitoring; (*g*) $Paco_2$

to the effects of these drugs. The frontalis muscle is less sensitive than the hypothenar muscles. Edmonds *et al.*[3] measured persistent EMG activity even during periods of hypothenar activity depression greater than 70%. Frontalis muscle activity can be used, although cautiously, in the presence of muscle relaxants. The EMG also rises artefactually, by changing the position of the patients, tracheal intubation or electrocoagulation.

The EMG increases after painful afferent stimuli during inadequate anaesthesia, and decreases again after the administration of an analgesic (*Figure 10.5*). Awakening and regaining of consciousness are always combined with a sudden increase in EMG irrespective of the type of anaesthetic. During the low spontaneous EMG periods, none of the subjects or patients was awake or not unconscious.

The zero crossing frequency decreases and the mean integrated voltage increases during intravenous induction of anaesthesia. When anaesthesia is maintained by an infusion of propofol, the zero crossing frequency regains its original value. When

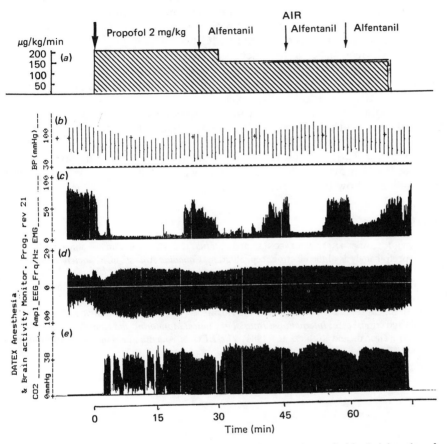

Figure 10.5 Example of inadequate anaesthesia level (from top to bottom): (*a*) administration of propofol and alfentanil; (*b*) systolic and diastolic blood pressures (lines) and heart rate (dots); (*c*) spontaneous EMG; (*d*) EEG: zero crossing frequency, above 0 line; mean integrated voltage, under 0 line; (*e*) Paco$_2$

anaesthesia is maintained with an inhalational anaesthetic, a transient rise in the zero crossing frequency occurs during the first 15 minutes. Benzodiazepines cause a rise in zero crossing frequency. These results are comparable with other studies[4]. As long as the combined spontaneous EMG value remains low, the zero crossing frequency increase does not indicate impending arousal. Not only the drug, but also the concentration, is important. Increasing the partial pressure in an inhalational anaesthetic results in a lower zero crossing frequency. There is an almost linear inverse relationship between blood propofol concentrations and the zero crossing frequency.

These relationships between zero crossing frequency and responses are less clearcut for the mean integrated voltage. An increase is noticed after induction.

This application was reliable only for early detection of cerebral hypo- or hyperactivity[5]. None of these changes of zero crossing frequency and mean integrated voltage correlated with awareness or unconsciousness.

The amplitude changes are moderate at the end of the procedure; the zero crossing frequency increases whatever the anaesthetic technique. Despite this increase, it is not possible to predict if the patient is already awake. The moment of awakening is, however, well seen on the EMG trace.

These new devices process the electrical activity of the brain, and of the spontaneous frontalis muscle, into qualitative and quantitative signals. The EEG parameters are dependent on anaesthetic agents and concentrations. They provide good warning of drug overdose or hypoxia.

The EMG values correlate well with unconsciousness or awareness during physiological sleep and anaesthesia. Absolute values are difficult to interpret, but the authors suggest that low EMG values correspond to unconsciousness and that a sudden rise of the EMG, in the absence of artefacts, is a warning for pending arousal. The EMG provides information about whether the patient is asleep, and the EEG indicates how the patient is asleep.

References

1. BEREZOWSKYJ, J. L., McEWEN, J., ANDERSON, G. and JENKINS, L. C. (1976) A study of anaesthesia depth by power spectral analysis of the electroencephalogram. *Canadian Anaesthetists' Society Journal*, **23**, 1–8

2. KAY, B. (1984) The anaesthesia and brain monitor (ABM). Concept and performance. *Acta Anaesthesiologica Belgica*, **35** (Suppl.), 167–174

3. EDMONDS, H. L., COUTURE, L. J., STOLZY, S. L. and PALOHEIMO, M. (1986) Quantitative surface EMG in anaesthesia and critical care. *International Journal of Clinical Monitoring and Computing*, **3**, 135–145

4. PICHLMAYR, I., LIPS, U. and KÜNKEL, H. (1984) *The EEG in Anaesthesia: Fundamentals, Practical Applications, Examples*. New York: Springer Verlag

5. EDMONDS, H. L. and PALOHEIMO, M. (1985) Computerized monitoring of the EMG and EEG during anesthesia. *International Journal of Clinical Monitoring and Computing*, **1**, 201–210

Chapter 11

Surface electromyography during low vigilance states

H. L. Edmonds Jr, S. L. Stolzy and L. J. Couture

Surface electromyography (surface EMG) provides the algebraic summation of electrical activity in a population of muscle fibres. There is a direct relationship between the integrated surface EMG amplitude and muscle tension during isometric muscle contraction (no movement)[1]. In drug-free conscious subjects, high tonic surface EMG amplitude is positively correlated with the level of motivation[2], vigilance[3] or psychological stress[4]. Phasic increases in amplitude are associated with periods of somatic stress, for example pain[5]. However, the relationship in drug states is less certain. Lader and Mathews[1] found that sedative agents which decreased vigilance did not necessarily reduce tonic surface EMG amplitude. Furthermore, it is difficult to determine unequivocally the cause of phasic surface EMG increases observed in anaesthetized or comatose patients.

The authors are investigating the causes of increased surface EMG activity during low level vigilance to clarify these relationships. The investigations include both drug and non-drug states in the evaluation of sleeping, comatose and anaesthetized patients. The ultimate goal of the study is to determine the clinical utility of surface EMG monitoring in unconscious patients.

Surface EMG measurements were made on the frontalis muscle, which has a relatively fixed length, to minimize the influence of the potentially confounding variable of changing fibre length (isotonic contraction). This muscle was chosen also because of its innervation by the special visceral efferent fibres of the facial nerve. The integrated surface EMG amplitude of the frontalis muscle provided a simple non-invasive measure of one aspect of autonomic tone. Voluntary and involuntary contractions of the frontalis muscle are innervated by separate pathways[6] and, therefore, the influence of volitional activity was minimized by monitoring unconscious patients. Since tonic (baseline) and phasic (abruptly increased) surface EMG activities may be differentially affected by altered levels of vigilance[7] or neuromuscular blocking agents[8], both components were quantified. The distinction is no longer made between spontaneous and evoked surface EMGs[9], because 'spontaneous' may indicate only that the nature of the evoking stimulus cannot be defined. So far, four evoking stimuli have been investigated: altered level of vigilance, altered emotional state, acoustic activation, and cerebral ischaemia. The surface EMG response to each of these evoking stimuli will be discussed separately.

Methods of recording and data analysis

Detailed descriptions of the recording technique used by the authors have been previously published[9,10]. Briefly, a complex biopotential is obtained from adhesive skin electrodes placed over the frontalis muscle and mastoid process (the indifferent electrode over the temporal bone). The biopotential is amplified, filtered, rectified and integrated with respect to time each second by a Datex/Puritan-Bennett Anaesthesia and Brain activity Monitor (ABM). The averages of successive 10-second intervals of integrated surface EMGs are displayed graphically on a semilogarithmic scale (*Figure 11.1*). For precise quantification, the output of the analogue-to-digital converter (ADC) used to generate the display was employed.

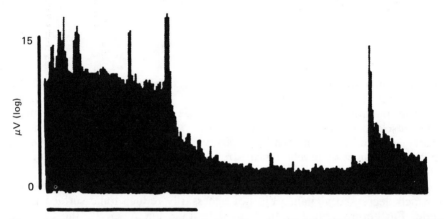

Figure 11.1 The progressive decrease in tonic frontalis surface EMG amplitude is shown on this ABM tracing during the change from wakefulness (trace above time marker) to deep slow wave sleep (middle of trace). Note the later increase (right portion of trace) associated with a period of apparently heightened vigilance. The horizontal bar in this and all subsequent figures represents a 15-min interval

The 65–400 Hz frequency band obtained from the broad band biopotential was normally used to provide an estimation of surface EMG activity. However, in some studies, the dynamic range was increased to 30–400 Hz by altering the high-pass filter design. The surface EMG amplitude scaling of the ABM graphic display was 0–15 µV or 0–255, from the ADC output. The dynamic range was increased four-fold by the stepwise addition of an attenuator to the pre-amplifier. This attenuation was necessary to quantify accurately the high levels of surface EMG that occur in surgical patients recovering from anaesthesia.

The digitized values of 10-second epochs of mean integrated surface EMG amplitude were recorded on digital tape. Data were then transferred to floppy disks for off-line statistical analysis by a Hewlett-Packard Model 216 computer and associated software.

Altered level of vigilance

Sleep

Minute-by-minute sleep stage determinations (hypnograms) based on visual interpretation of polygraphic recordings were made by an experienced electroencephalographer[11]. The surface EMG, associated with the activity of frontalis and other scalp muscles, was recorded by the ABM using the P_4–O_2 EEG electrode pair. This unusual posterior derivation minimized the influences of eye movement or deep breathing on the surface EMG amplitude. It also resulted in an attenuated signal that prevented pre-amplifier saturation during periods of high vigilance.

In all sleep stages, the frontalis activity was low relative to wakefulness, and there were no statistically significant stage-related differences in surface EMG amplitude. Therefore, the mean amplitude during wakefulness was compared to that in the non-waking state in seven sleep-deprived patients with suspected idiopathic epilepsy.

The average non-waking surface EMG was 34% (s.d. = 20) ($P < 0.015$ by paired Student's t, two-tailed) of the waking value. *Figure 11.1* illustrates the depression in surface EMG amplitude during the progression from wakefulness to sleep and the subsequent phasic increase during periods of heightened vigilance. These data indicate that although frontalis surface EMG alone is insufficient for sleep staging, it can discriminate between wakefulness and non-wakefulness in the non-drug state. This simple technique may thus prove useful in the diagnosis of sleep disorders. Its application for the objective assessment of hypnotic drug efficacy must await additional verification.

Anaesthesia

The lowering of vigilance accompanying induction of general anaesthesia is typically associated with dramatic decreases in tonic frontalis activity. Several groups[8,10,12,13] concluded that phasic increases in this drug-induced surface EMG amplitude depression are indicative of inadequate anaesthesia. Further, all these investigators observed that phasic surface EMG increases could occur in the presence of neuromuscular blocking agents.

In 15 ASA grade I–III surgical patients (ASA = American Society of Anesthesiologists) the changes in frontalis activity were examined during the progression from wakefulness to profound surgical anaesthesia. A standardized and carefully controlled isoflurane-based anaesthetic protocol was used to minimize the influence of extraneous variables[14]. Surface EMG amplitude in the median 10-second pre-induction epoch was compared with the surface EMGs obtained 1 minute before and during the initial surgical incision. The relationship between the magnitude of the latter phasic change to the end-tidal isoflurane concentration was also determined.

Figure 11.2 depicts the rapid decrease in tonic frontalis surface EMG amplitude that typically occurs during the diminished vigilance induced by barbiturates[15]. Note the subsequent increase during tracheal intubation, which is suggestive of an inadequate anaesthetic effect. Immediately before the surgical stimulus, the tonic surface EMG logarithm of the amplitude had decreased 86% (s.d. = 9) from the pre-induction baseline ($P < 0.001$). Because of the relatively high dose of isoflurane (1.5–2.5%), detectable phasic increases in surface EMG amplitude associated with surgical stimulation did not occur.

Because of wide variability in the nature of the subsequent surgical stimuli and total minimum alveolar concentration/hour exposure, surface EMG changes occurring during recovery were examined in a separate study involving 21 additional patients. A somewhat different, but equally standardized, isoflurane-

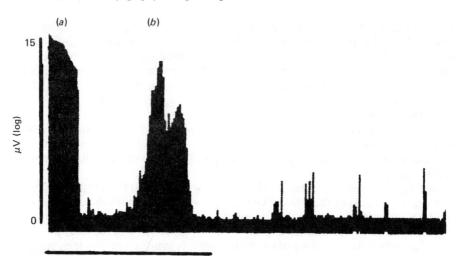

Figure 11.2 A rapid decrease in tonic frontalis muscle activity (*a*) typically occurs during induction of anaesthesia with thiopentone. Infrequently, phasic increases in surface EMG amplitude may be seen during intubation (*b*). Such increases are not usually due to movement artefact but rather seem to indicate an inadequate anaesthetic effect

based anaesthetic protocol was used[16]. However, the surgical stimulus (arthroscopy) and minimum alveolar concentration/hour exposure were kept as constant as possible in a clinical study of this type.

The mean surface EMG amplitude and coefficient of variation were determined in three successive 15-minute intervals following the patient's admission to the recovery room. The relationship between changes in surface EMG amplitude and activity score (measure of vigilance) was examined by linear regression. In addition, the association of phasic surface increases with verbal indications of pain was determined.

Within the first hour after the patient's admission to the recovery room, the mean amplitude of tonic frontalis activity was commonly well above values observed earlier in anaesthetized patients. In addition, there was a significant correlation between mean surface EMG amplitude and activity score ($r = 0.54$, 19 degrees of freedom, $P < 0.025$). There was a time-related increase in the coefficient of variation of the surface EMG amplitude indicating increased variability associated with a rising state of vigilance. These findings are consistent with the authors' earlier observations[17].

Altered emotional state

Results obtained in the above study on post-operative pain indicate that large amplitude phasic increases in surface EMGs were associated with the patient's unmistakable verbal expression of marked and persistent discomfort. Of 43 patients who demonstrated phasic increases larger than 50% of the baseline, 31 were coupled with evidence of pain ($P < 0.05$ by chi-square, one-tailed).

Emotion-related changes in surface EMG amplitude have also been observed in comatose patients. In the absence of central depressant or paralysing drugs, phasic bursts of frontalis activity following painful stimulation can be demonstrated in

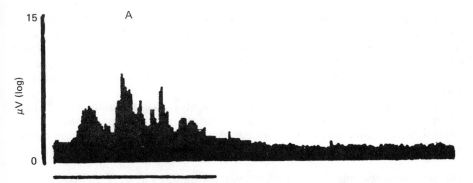

Figure 11.3 This recording was made from a head trauma patient with a Glasgow coma score of 8. The tracing depicts a phasic increase in frontalis surface EMG in response to electrical stimulation (marker A) (train-of-four square wave pulses with 70 mA current at 20-s intervals) of the ulnar nerve. Such phasic responses to painful stimuli have often been observed in patients with a moderately depressed level of vigilance

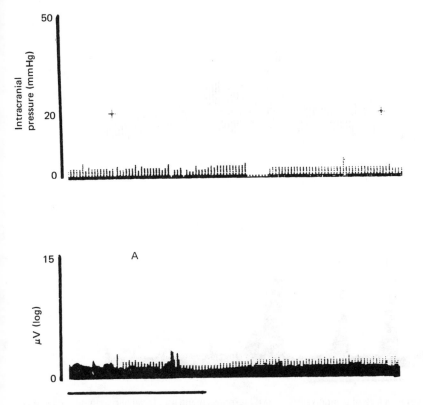

Figure 11.4 At marker (A), train-of-four facial nerve stimulation in a head-injured patient with a Glasgow coma score of 3 shows an absence of response in both the frontalis muscle and intracranial pressure. This unresponsiveness is typical for patients with a severely depressed level of vigilance

moderately comatose (Glasgow coma score 6–8) patients. *Figure 11.3* illustrates the surface EMG response to electrical stimulation (train-of-four, 2-Hz 0.1-ms square wave pulses with 70 mA current presented at 20-second intervals) of the ulnar nerve. In such patients, the magnitude of the surface EMG response to the standardized electrical stimulus provides a convenient and objective measure of reactivity.

In contrast, unmedicated deeply comatose patients (Glasgow coma score <6) are typically unresponsive to the painful electrical stimulation (*Figure 11.4*). Nevertheless, auditory stimuli with a high affective content (talking from family member) can occasionally elicit dramatic phasic surface EMG responses (*Figure 11.5*).

The persistent response of the pain-activated frontalis surface EMG response in deeply comatose patients is atypical. Recently, this pattern was observed in a patient whose obtunded state was due to an undiagnosed drug overdose rather than to cerebral trauma (*Figure 11.6*). Haemodialysis reversed the coma in this individual who had been diagnosed as having severe brain injury.

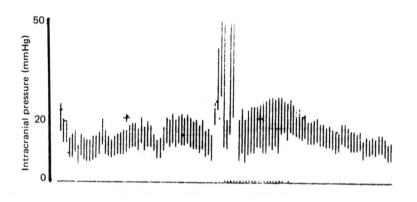

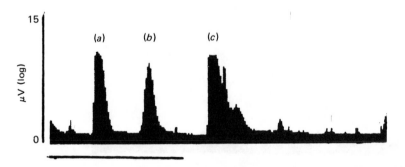

Figure 11.5 Despite a lack of frontalis surface EMG response to ulnar or facial nerve stimulation in this deeply comatose patient, phasic increases were observed in response to comments from a family member (*a*) and an investigator (*b*). Note the relatively stable intracranial pressure during these events (upper trace). At (*c*) tracheal suction led to increases in both surface EMG and intracranial pressure

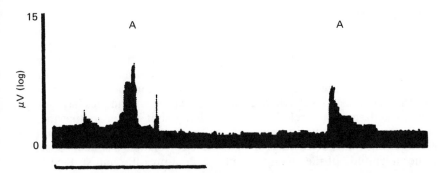

Figure 11.6 Phasic frontalis surface EMG activity in response to painful stimulation (A) was observed in a patient thought to have severe brain injury as the result of post-traumatic convulsions. Since such phasic stimulus-evoked responses are unusual during deep coma, an alternative diagnosis was sought. The potentially depressant influence of aggressive anticonvulsant therapy was minimized by haemodialysis. During this procedure, the patient regained consciousness and was ultimately discharged from the hospital with no apparent residual deficit

Acoustic activation

There are a variety of causes for the acoustically evoked phasic increases in frontalis surface EMG amplitude. Both the frontalis and stapedius muscles are innervated by special visceral efferent fibres of the facial nerve. Simultaneous activation of both these muscles occurs in response to a sudden loud noise (acousticofacial reflex). Normal intensity sound also results in dampening of the auditory ossicles by the stapedius. Even in deeply anaesthetized patients, the authors have observed phasic surface EMG activity associated with this acoustic input (*Figure 11.7*). In the absence of a significant relationship between end-tidal anaesthetic gas concentration and phasic surface EMG amplitude, a contribution from the cochlear microphonic or its summating potential cannot be entirely excluded. However, recording from cadavers did show that the response was not due simply to electrode vibration.

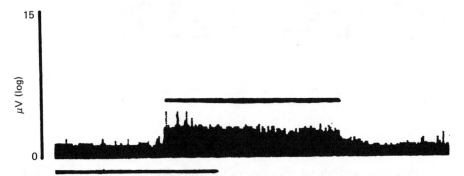

Figure 11.7 A tape-recorded message, at an intensity of approximately 60 phons, was presented to deeply anaesthetized patients (horizontal bar over trace). Phasic increases in frontalis surface EMG coincident with such acoustic stimulation were typically observed, although the precise cause of the increase has yet to be determined

Cerebral ischaemia

Elevated intracranial pressure can result in cerebral ischaemia. Inadequate cerebral perfusion triggers a reflex activation of the cerebrovasodilator nerve fibres, which are also innervated by the facial nerve[18,19]. The relationship between phasic increases in intracranial pressure and surface EMG have thus been examined. An example of this relationship is shown in *Figure 11.8*. Sufficient samples have not yet been obtained to describe the relationship completely, but it appears that the first time derivatives of these two parameters are linearly related. Although their absolute magnitudes do not co-vary, a significant correlation has been observed between the magnitude of the changes in intracranial pressure and surface EMG over time during periods of carefully controlled and documented environmental conditions.

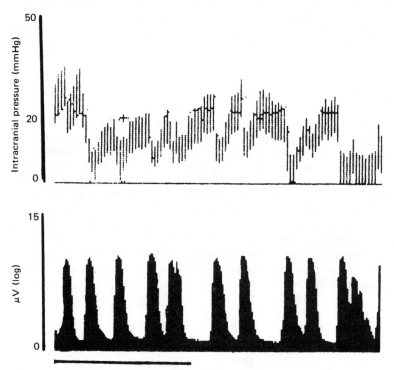

Figure 11.8 In addition to activating influences of pain (*Figure 11.6*), emotional stress (*Figure 11.5*) or sound (*Figure 11.7*), transient elevations in intracranial pressure can also elicit phasic surface EMG increases of frontalis activity. This figure illustrates the close association between increases in surface EMG and intracranial pressure in a head-injured comatose patient

Conclusions

It appears that tonic and phasic activities of the frontalis muscle are differentially innervated and responsive to anaesthetic or relaxant agents. However, the integrated surface EMG criteria for tonic and phasic activities are somewhat arbitrary so that an unambiguous distinction between the two is not always possible. For example, in comatose patients apparent phasic increases in frontalis surface EMG, persisting for many hours, may be superimposed on a persistent low amplitude baseline of tonic activity. Nevertheless, there seems to be a direct relationship between apparent tonic frontalis surface EMG amplitude and level of vigilance if the full range of behaviours from conscious agitation to profound anaesthesia or coma is examined. Thus, the authors' findings are not inconsistent with the limited vigilance range examined earlier by Lader and Mathews[1].

It has been demonstrated that at least three fundamentally different types of physiological stimuli – emotion, sound and ischaemia – may evoke a phasic increase in surface EMG amplitude during low vigilance states. Therefore, careful documentation and control of environmental changes, e.g. auditory stimuli, are necessary to accurately interpret phasic surface EMG changes.

Acknowledgements

The authors are grateful for Datex Instrumentarium and the Puritan-Bennett Corporation for supplying the monitors and computers used in these studies and to Dr B. M. Rigor Sr for his continued advice and support.

References

1. LADER, M. H. and MATHEWS, A. M. (1971) Electromyographic studies of tension. *Journal of Psychosomatic Research*, **15**, 479–486
2. SURWILLO, W. W. (1956) Psychological factors in muscle-action potentials: EMG gradients. *Journal of Experimental Psychology*, **52**, 263–272
3. KENNEDY, J. L. and TRAVIS, R. C. (1947) Prediction of speed of performance by muscle action potentials. *Science*, **105**, 410–411
4. MALMO, R. B. and SMITH, A. A. (1955) Forehead tension and motor irregularities in psychoneurotic patients under stress. *Journal of Personality*, **23**, 391–406
5. BUDZYNSKI, T., STOYVA, J. and ADLER, C. (1970) Feedback-induced muscle relaxation: application to tension headache. *Journal of Behavior Therapy and Experimental Psychiatry*, **1**, 205–211
6. TRUEX, R. G. and CARPENTER, M. B. (1969) *Human Neuroanatomy*, pp. 356–360. Baltimore: Williams & Wilkins
7. DEMENT, W. and KLEITMAN, N. (1957) The relation of eye movements during sleep to dream activity: an objective method for the study of dreaming. *Journal of Experimental Psychology*, **53**, 339–346
8. EDMONDS, H. L. JR, TRIANTAFILLOU, T., TSUEDA, I. and PALOHEIMO, M. (1985) Comparison of frontalis and hypothenar EMG responses to vecuronium. *Anesthesiology*, **63**, A324
9. EDMONDS, H. L. JR, COUTURE, L. J., STOLZY, S. L. and PALOHEIMO, M. (1986) Quantitative surface electromyography in anesthesia and critical care. *International Journal of Clinical Monitoring and Computing*, **3**, 135–145
10. EDMONDS, H. L. JR and PALOHEIMO, M. (1985) Computerized monitoring of the EMG and EEG during anesthesia: an evaluation of the Anesthesia and Brain activity Monitor (ABM). *International Journal of Clinical Monitoring and Computing*, **1**, 201–210
11. EDMONDS, H. L. JR, DECLERCK, A. C. and WAUQUIER, A. (1985) Level of consciousness as determined by combined EEG frequency and amplitude analysis. *International Journal of Clinical Monitoring and Computing*, **1**, 75
12. HARMEL, M. H., KLEIN, F. F. and DAVIS, D. A. (1978) The EEMG – a practical index of cortical activity and muscular relaxation. *Acta Anaesthesiologica Scandinavica Supplementum*, **70**, 97–102
13. WATT, R. C., HAMEROFF, S. R., CORK, R. C., CALKINS, J. M., KEYS, C. A. and MYLREA, K. C. (1985) Spontaneous EMG monitoring for anesthetic depth assessment. *Proceedings of the Association of Advanced Medical Instrumentation*, **20**, 92
14. COUTURE, L. J., STOLZY, S. L. and EDMONDS, H. L. JR (1986) EMG response to auditory stimuli under isoflurane anesthesia. *Anesthesia and Analgesia*, **65**, S36

15. MARTIN, I. and DAVIES, B. M. (1965) The effect of sodium amytal on autonomic and muscle activity in patients with depressive illness. *British Journal of Psychiatry,* **111**, 168–175
16. EDMONDS, H. L. JR, RIGOR, B. M., DEMPSEY, F. J. and SHEA, R. G . (1986) A double-blind comparison of fentanyl and butorphanol as adjuncts during arthroscopy. *Proceedings of the 7th European Congress of Anaesthesiology* **17**, 342
17. EDMONDS, H. L. JR, BUCK, J. S., TSUEDA, K. and RIGOR, B. M. (1985) Assessment of postoperative analgesia by the computerized spontaneous electromyogram. *International Journal of Clinical Monitoring and Computing,* **1**, 282
18. CHOROBSKI, J. and PENFIELD, W. (1932) Cerebral vasodilator nerves and their pathway from the medulla oblongata, with observations on pial and intracerebral vascular plexus. *Archives of Neurology and Psychiatry,* **28**, 1257–1289
19. EDVINSSON, L. (1975) Neurogenic mechanisms in the cerebrovascular bed. Autonomic nerves, amine receptors and their effects on cerebral blood flow. *Acta Physiologica Scandinavica Supplementum,* **427**, 1–35

Chapter 12

Use of evoked responses in the EEG to measure depth of anaesthesia

J. G. Jones

The term 'depth of anaesthesia' is defined here as the functional state of the brain which results from an interaction between the excitatory effects of surgical stimulation and the depressant effects of anaesthetic action on endogenous cerebral activity.

The clinical assessment of the functional state of the brain during anaesthesia depends largely on signs of autonomic activity, such as sweating, tears or changing heart rate, blood pressure and pupil size. It must be admitted, however, that it is not easy to judge depth of anaesthesia using these criteria, and most anaesthetists rely on their past experience in judging the amount and type of anaesthetic required to keep the patient unconscious. This is because these changes in autonomic function are not particularly good indicators of depth of anaesthesia due to individual differences in autonomic responses to surgical stimulation and the concomitant use of drugs that may attenuate these responses[1]. Occasionally, a retrospective assessment of brain function is made post-operatively when the patient is questioned about mental function or recall of events that occurred during the operation[2]. Some patients, so lightly anaesthetized that they were able to respond to commands to open or close their fingers, had no recollection of these commands on recovery from anaesthesia[3]. Other patients describe having 'dreams' in which they may remember some intra-operative events and this may imply a light level of anaesthesia. In rare circumstances, intra-operative events may be recalled with such graphic detail that it is evident that the patient was wide awake during the operative procedure and this was not recognized at the time because the patient had been given a neuromuscular blocking drug and because autonomic signs were not noticed or did not change significantly[4]. At the other extreme some patients may not regain consciousness at the end of an anaesthetic, and it is only then realized that brain damage had occurred but was unrecognized during anaesthesia.

More recently, there is increasing evidence that anaesthetized patients may recall word lists 'heard' whilst anaesthetized or whose behaviour may be modified by their being given audible instructions during their anaesthetic[5-7]. These patients were judged to have been satisfactorily anaesthetized based on the criterion of a generally acceptable concentration of anaesthetic being delivered to the patient at the time.

These observations justify closer attention to the question of monitoring depth of anaesthesia during surgery and raise a number of problems which have not yet been solved. These problems are:

- Measuring graded effects of anaesthetics on the brain.
- Recognizing the fully conscious but paralysed patient.
- Hearing and memory in apparently anaesthetized patients.
- Evaluation of brain injury during anaesthesia.

The requirements for quantification of the functional state of the brain during anaesthesia would include the following:

- An easily produced signal which provides an objective measurement of depth of anaesthesia.
- The signal should be unaffected by muscle relaxants.
- All general anaesthetic drugs should give similar changes in the signal.
- The signal should be sensitive to brain injury.

Approaches to the assessment of brain function during anaesthesia

The brain is a highly active metabolic organ whose function may be assessed either in terms of its specialized neuronal activity, blood flow, metabolic activity and electrical activity.

Specialized neuronal activity

The prime effect of general anaesthesia is to impair specialized neuronal function such as consciousness, memory, motor responses to sensory stimulation, and autonomic control. Consequently, the conventional clinical methods for assessing function of the CNS are useless, especially in patients treated with neuromuscular blocking drugs.

Cerebral blood flow

Regional cerebral blood flow is very closely matched to regional cerebral metabolism, so it is possible to derive an index of metabolism from changes in regional blood flow. However, under the very circumstances that we may wish to assess brain metabolism, that is during anaesthesia or after a head injury, the normal close link between flow and metabolism is broken[8]. Thus, the demonstration of a reduced blood flow may be useful in identifying the cause of brain injury, but most volatile anaesthetics and injury itself may result in a higher blood flow than would be expected from a particular level of brain metabolism.

Cerebral metabolism

Measurements of brain metabolism may be made in a number of ways during anaesthesia. If the gradients of oxygen or glucose across the brain are measured simultaneously with cerebral blood flow, the cerebral metabolic rate for oxygen or glucose can be calculated. This gives information about the metabolism of the whole brain, but cannot detect changes in metabolism of discrete regions. Regional cerebral metabolism can be determined in three ways: regional uptake of radiolabelled glucose using autoradiography in animals; positron emission tomography in man and magnetic resonance spectroscopy.

Some of these beautiful imaging techniques show that brain cell metabolism is very non-uniform in different parts of the brain and is highly correlated with brain cell function in health and disease. However, none of them can be used for routine monitoring in the operating room. Nevertheless, they all provide invaluable information about regional brain function and regional sites of action of anaesthetics in the brain, and are invaluable correlates of electrophysiological techniques which are the only methods so far applicable in the operating room.

Electrical activity

Until the recent development of imaging techniques, most of our knowledge of neurophysiology had been derived from studies of electrical activity from within discrete parts of the brain. The electroencephalogram (EEG) derived using electrodes placed on the surface of the scalp gives some information about regional function of the cortex in man.

The EEG represents the metabolic activity used for the specialized neuronal, rather than the basal, function of the cell. For example, the EEG is depressed in localized or global ischaemia, narcosis or hypothermia when the specialized neuronal function is depressed[9]. The EEG becomes isoelectric when mean arterial pressure falls to between 20 and 40 mmHg and cerebral blood flow to 18–24 ml/min per 100 g. Prior (Chapter 5) has reviewed the effects of general anaesthesia on the EEG and has described quite different effects of different anaesthetics on this complex signal. This makes the unprocessed EEG unattractive for the clinician who is looking for an unambiguous signal to demonstrate graded changes in depth of anaesthesia. Consequently, the need for an easily interpreted signal, which could also be used in feedback control of the administration of anaesthetics, led to the study of the processed EEG signal.

The processed EEG as an indicator of anaesthetic depth

Prior points out (Chapter 5) that the traditional methods for electronic analysis of the EEG have quantified events either in the frequency domain or in the time domain. The former, measuring voltage or power against frequency[10,11] has been used for a number of years, but more recently attention has focused on two parts of this domain – the spectral edge frequency and median frequency.

The spectral edge frequency

This is the frequency below which lies 95% of the power in the processed EEG. Spectral edge frequency normally has a value of about 25 Hz in awake man and animals and a progressive fall in spectral edge frequency occurs with increasing concentrations of halothane, enflurane[12], thiopentone[13], etomidate[14], fentanyl and alfentanil[15]. All of these studies showed a close relationship between the reduction in spectral edge frequency and increasing levels of anaesthetic drug during the transition between the awake state and stage 2 anaesthesia. However, this is not a useful technique for measuring depth of anaesthesia because, during the transition phase from deep to light levels of anaesthesia, the relationship between spectral edge frequency and blood level of the anaesthetic was very poor[14]. In contrast, the same group[14] found that the median EEG frequency showed a much better correlation with drug level, both in the uptake and elimination phases. The explanation for the close relationship between spectral edge frequency and blood levels during light stages of anaesthesia was based on the spectral edge frequency being more sensitive than median frequency to an EEG power spectrum skewed by high frequency (>13 Hz) waves seen with arousal and anxiety. These features are more likely during uptake than elimination of anaesthetic.

The median frequency

This is discussed by Stoeckel and Schwilden[16] (*see* Chapter 7). They show fairly consistent correlations of the median frequency with plasma concentration of etomidate and with clinical signs of different stages of anaesthesia, e.g. awake, falling asleep, lack of response to command, loss of lid reflex and then corneal reflex. However, the EEG median frequency at full orientation was lower than pre-anaesthetic values which may pose a problem if median frequency is used as a guide to anaesthetic depth. It must be emphasized that expressing all the information in the EEG by a single number may be misleading, because many different frequency distributions, having quite different clinical implications, may have the same median frequency[11,17] (Prior, personal communication).

Time domain analysis includes the cerebral function monitor (CFM) and cerebral function analysing monitor (CFAM) both of which are discussed by Frank and Prior (Chapter 8), and various evoked potentials in the EEG.

Evoked potentials

These are electrical responses of the nervous system which are locked in time (or phase) to a variety of stimuli which induce them. The nervous system is constantly generating potentials because of its endogenous activity, and this is easily recorded from scalp electrodes. An evoked potential is an electrical manifestation of the brain response to an external stimulus[18]. The visual evoked potential produced by a flash of light can be seen as a wave in the EEG measured over the occipital region. In contrast, evoked potentials produced from discrete auditory or somatic stimuli may be 100 times smaller than the 'noise' of the spontaneous EEG and can rarely be recorded without signal averaging.

Three steps are necessary to produce an evoked potential[19]: a brief stimulus; a record of the electrical response of the nervous system; and elimination of background noise.

The stimuli used to generate evoked potentials are either visual, tactile or auditory, although responses have been elicited to a number of other stimuli including olfactory, thermal or gustatory stimuli. A repetitive stimulus evokes a series of potentials in the EEG, which are aligned to the time that the stimulus starts and are then summed together.

An evoked potential always comes at the same interval after the stimulus, in contrast to the background electrical activity which is not stimulus coupled. The time locked evoked potential is repeatedly summed as the stimulus is repeated and other electrical activity is gradually eliminated by the averaging procedure.

This process of signal averaging produces one or more electrical potentials each of which may be generated by a specific anatomical structure and its interconnections within the brain. The exact spatial resolution of the origins of evoked potentials is not possible because of the disturbing effects of volume conduction within the brain on the electrical signal. A major improvement in spatial resolving power is achieved using neuromagnetic fields measured with a superconducting quantum interference device (SQUID)[20]. However, these devices are much more complicated and expensive than evoked potentials and have not yet been used to study the effects of anaesthesia.

One of the important technical aspects of producing good quality evoked potentials is the electrode type and position which is discussed by Regan[21] and Halliday[22]. The 10–20 electrode system of placement on the scalp is almost universally employed. For example, a line designated z, from nasion to inion is divided into five points: frontal pole (FP), frontal (F), central (C), parietal (P) and occipital (O). The frontal pole is 10% of the nasion–inion distance above the nasion, frontal is 20% of this distance back from frontal pole and so on in 20% steps for central, parietal and occipital (thus the 10–20 system). The scalp is divided similarly for non-midline positions giving a total of 21 electrode positions. The electrode position for different evoked potentials and different latencies are described in the specialized texts mentioned above.

An outline of the cardinal features of visual, somatosensory and auditory evoked potentials will be given in the following section.

Visual evoked potentials

Action potentials, set up in the retina by a light stimulus, pass along the optic nerves to the lateral geniculate bodies and thence to the cortical cells. The stimulus employed is usually the reversing chequer-board pattern of light which is arranged so that the squares reverse colour without a change in total light output. Alternatively, a flash stimulus may be employed which changes the light level falling on the retina and produces a much greater range of variation in the visual evoked potential than with the chequer-board stimulus. The chequer-board pattern is reversed about 1–2 times per second and the visual evoked potential is produced by signal averaging. The normal visual evoked potential (occipital referred to Fz) is dominated by a large positive wave with a latency of 100 ms (P_{100}) generated in the striate and parastriate visual cortex. In addition to the P_{100}, there are much less prominent waves with either shorter or longer latency. The standard deviation of the latency of the P_{100} is only 4 ms and the stability of its position accounts for its usefulness. The amplitude and latency of P_{100} depends upon the integrity of the visual pathway which may be impaired by pathological processes, surgery or the effects of drugs. Flash visual evoked potentials show large intersubject variation but are useful for studying changes in any given subject[18].

Somatosensory evoked potentials

The stimulus is usually a percutaneous electrical stimulation of a peripheral nerve, although tapping or even blowing puffs of air on the skin may be employed. Sensing electrodes may be placed over the brachial plexus (Erb's point), cervical spine or scalp and, with electrodes at these locations, the transmission of the stimulating wave through the nervous system is well demonstrated. Thus, the somatosensory evoked potential waveform depends upon electrode position and whether an upper or lower limb nerve is being stimulated. Subcortical or spinal potentials are often referred to as 'far field' and cortical as 'near field' potentials[23]. There is a close relationship between the waveform and the anatomy of the sensory tracts, particularly in far field potentials. The morphology of far field potentials is relatively insensitive to changing electrode position, whereas near field potentials are very sensitive to electrode position. The electrical stimulus is a square wave of 0.2–2 ms duration, the optimal rate of stimulation being 5 per s with faster rates causing changes in latency and amplitude[18]. After stimulation of the median nerve, waves are seen between 11 and 13 ms (N11, N13, P13) which correspond to ascending volleys in the posterior column of the cervical cord and dorsal column nuclei. The earliest potential of cortical origin is a negative wave with a latency of 20 ms (the N1, or N20 wave). There is a positive wave at 25 ms, a negative wave at 30 ms and a large positive wave at 40 ms. By measuring the time between the spinal potential (N13) and the first cortical component (N20), the conduction velocity of the sensory pathways can be calculated.

Auditory evoked responses

Auditory stimuli are delivered via headphones which provide a series of clicks or tone bursts. The frequency and intensity of the sound can be varied. A 6-Hz stimulating frequency has been used in all the authors' studies of the auditory evoked response. The click intensity is adjusted to 70 dB above the hearing threshold. Decreased stimulus intensity produces longer latency and a decrease in amplitude particularly of waves II–IV. The first 10 ms (*Figure 12.1*) of the response arises from the brainstem (far field potentials); from 10 to 100 ms (*Figure 12.2*), the middle latency response arises from the primary auditory cortex[24] and

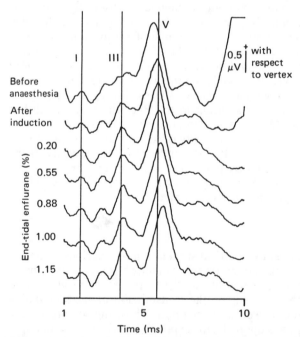

Figure 12.1 Averaged brainstem auditory evoked response for one subject, before anaesthesia, following induction and at different concentrations of end-tidal enflurane (vol. %). A vertical line indicates the position of waves I, III and V at the lowest enflurane concentration. (Reproduced by permission of the authors and publishers of the *British Journal of Anaesthesia*[26])

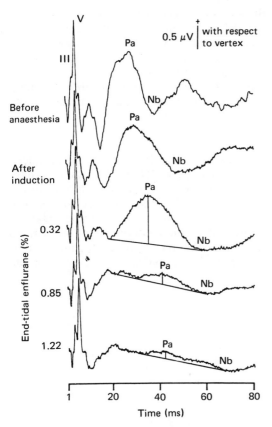

Figure 12.2 Averaged early cortical auditory evoked response for one subject, before anaesthesia, following induction and at different concentrations of end-tidal enflurane (vol. %). Amplitude measurements of Pa indicated by vertical line. (Reproduced by permission of the authors and publishers of the *British Journal of Anaesthesia*[26])

hippocampus; the response with latencies longer than 100 ms arises from cortical association areas (near field potentials). The amplitude of the waves tends to be maximal at the vertex (Cz location). A steady-state auditory potential, rather than a transient response, may be recorded using a 40-Hz signal[25]. This frequency is close to the frequency of the principal waves in the middle latency response and is easy to record from normal subjects.

Effects of general anaesthesia on the evoked potential

Research at Northwick Park Hospital on evoked potentials has been confined to the auditory evoked responses and details of the technique have been previously published[26]. The majority of these studies were carried out before and after induction of anaesthesia with sodium thiopentone prior to the start of surgery, although the concluding section will discuss the effects of surgery on the evoked potential. The usual procedure for these investigations was as follows. Following a series of measurements of evoked potentials in patients paralysed with pancuronium and with the lungs ventilated with nitrous oxide and oxygen, one of the anaesthetic agents under test was added in increments, a suitable time being allowed at each increment to achieve a quasi-steady state. Particular care was taken in these studies to maintain a constant $Paco_2$ and body temperature because of the effects on the evoked potential of changes in these variables.

All these studies were carried out prior to the start of surgery and are subdivided into the effects on the brainstem potentials and effects on the early cortical (middle latency) potentials and can best be summarized as follows.

Brainstem effects
The volatile anaesthetics halothane, enflurane and isoflurane, all produced dose-related changes in the latency of brainstem waves III and V, although there was no change in amplitude of these waves. The graded effect of enflurane on the latency of waves III and V is shown in *Figure 12.1*. Other workers have shown similar effects on the latency of these brainstem waves of thiopentone (James, M.F.M., 1985, personal communication) and methohexitone[27]. In contrast, no effect on the brainstem latencies was seen with either nitrous oxide, the intravenous agents alphaxalone–alphadalone (Althesin)[28], etomidate[29] and the opioid

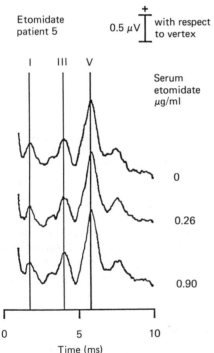

Figure 12.3 Shows the lack of effect of etomidate on the latency of brainstem waves[29]. In contrast, etomidate produces changes in the middle latency waves similar to those seen in *Figure 12.2*

fentanyl[30]. The lack of effect of etomidate on the brainstem latencies is shown in *Figure 12.3*. It is clear from these results that the changes in brainstem latencies do not provide a universal signal that could be used to demonstrate effects of graded anaesthetic action.

Cortical effects
Much more promising was the effect of all of these anaesthetics on the early cortical (middle latency) responses. In the authors' studies halothane, enflurane, isoflurane[26,31,32], Althesin, etomidate and propofol[32] all produced graded, dose-related changes in the amplitude of the early cortical responses. In particular the amplitudes of waves Pa, Nb and Pb were very sensitive to graded changes in anaesthetic concentrations (MAC = minimum alveolar concentration), and at concentrations equivalent to 1 MAC, waves Nb and Pb could not be identified (*Figure 12.2*). It seems that the longer the latency, the greater the susceptibility to anaesthetic action in terms of a reduction in wave amplitude, the amplitude of the brainstem waves showing no effect, whereas the middle latency waves are very susceptible.

The effects of decreasing anaesthetic concentrations on the auditory evoked responses has not been rigorously studied by the Northwick Park Group. Reducing halothane concentration reversed the effect both on brainstem latency and on the amplitude of the early cortical waves Pa, Nb and Pb[26]. A similar reversal of the effect on the latter waves was seen following a reduction in the rate of Althesin infusion[26].

Correlation between anaesthetic action on evoked potential and brain metabolism

The lack of effect of Althesin, etomidate and fentanyl on brainstem evoked responses in man was of particular interest in relation to other studies of regional differences in the metabolic effects of these anaesthetics. Davis and colleagues[34,35] and Young *et al.*[36] have shown a comparable sparing effect of Althesin, etomidate and sufentanil on brainstem metabolism in animals. In contrast, there is a reduction in cerebral metabolism of the brainstem and cortex with barbiturates, halothane and isoflurane[37,38]. Thus, two quite different techniques, evoked potentials and regional metabolism, in two different species, man and rat, produce evidence of comparable differences in anaesthetic action in the brain. Davis and colleagues[34,35] suggest that these differences may be due to different regional distribution of anaesthetic specific receptors for these agents within the brain. While this may not be a novel idea in the case of the opioid sufentanil, it is a fascinating concept in the case of the other two agents.

These findings focus attention on the amplitude of early cortical waves as the most promising signal with which to judge depth of anaesthesia. Furthermore, it suggests that anaesthetic action at the level of the cortex rather than the brainstem, at least up to the level of the inferior colliculus, is the site of anaesthetic action that best correlates with loss of consciousness. The greater sensitivity to anaesthetics of parts of the brain which generate waves whose latency is longer than 20 ms suggests that the function of cortical association areas, rather than that of the primary cortex, may be readily depressed by anaesthetic action.

Other workers have studied anaesthetic action on the evoked potentials in man. Sebel *et al.*[39] showed a dose-related effect of nitrous oxide on the amplitudes of visual evoked potentials and somatosensory evoked potentials, although there was no effect on brainstem auditory evoked potential. Uhl *et al.*[40] showed that halothane produced graded increases in latency of visual evoked potentials. Sebel *et al.*[41] showed that isoflurane, up to 1.65% end-tidal concentrations, produced dose-related changes in the amplitude and latencies of visual evoked potentials, somatosensory evoked potentials and brainstem auditory evoked potentials. They concluded that the most consistent results occurred with somatosensory evoked potentials. Peterson, Drummond and Todd[42] studied the effect of halothane, enflurane, isoflurane and nitrous oxide on the somatosensory evoked potentials and showed dose-related changes in amplitude and latency of the cortical components. These were most pronounced with enflurane and least with halothane.

The effect of surgical stimuli on auditory evoked responses

The results described so far show similar dose-related effects on the auditory evoked responses of halothane, enflurane, isoflurane, Althesin, etomidate and propofol in clinically relevant dosage. However, if a rapid means of measuring the blood levels of these drugs was available, the auditory evoked response would appear to provide, on the evidence so far presented, only a little more information than that provided by the drug level itself. Any differences would represent the well-known individual differences in susceptibility of the CNS to anaesthetic action, and the problem of predicting brain concentration of drugs from their blood concentration. The auditory evoked response would thus appear to be a bioassay of anaesthetic concentration. However, the concept of depth of anaesthesia described at the beginning of this chapter suggests a balance between the depressant effects of general anaesthetics and the stimulating effects of surgery on endogenous cerebral activity. If the auditory evoked response were to reflect this balance, it would have to be sensitive to changes in surgical stimulation as well as to anaesthetic concentration.

To examine this hypothesis, patients were anaesthetized with sodium thiopentone, paralysed in the usual way and with anaesthesia maintained with nitrous oxide, oxygen and 0.3% end-tidal halothane. When $Paco_2$ and core temperature were controlled at pre-anaesthetic levels, a series of auditory evoked responses were obtained during a 30-min baseline period. Then surgery commenced and, for a further 30-min period, a second series of auditory evoked responses was obtained. Autonomic responses were noted, such as changes in heart rate, blood pressure, pupillary reaction, sweating and lacrimation.

The results of this study revealed the following:

- During the baseline period, the wave Pb was absent from the auditory evoked response and there was a reduction in amplitude of Pa and Nb.
- During the period of surgical stimulation, eight out of the 11 patients showed a significant increase in amplitude of Pa, Nb and Pb.
- Three of the patients showed an increased autonomic response, but there was no relationship between increased autonomic activity and arousal in the auditory evoked response.

These results support the hypothesis that the middle latency of the auditory evoked response may be employed to measure depth of anaesthesia, in that it reflects both graded concentrations of anaesthetics and the effects of surgical stimuli. Other workers have reported a change in evoked potentials with change in conscious state. An increase in amplitude of long latencies in the auditory evoked response has been reported with awake subjects when attention is aroused by extraneous stimuli[43]. Angel et al.[44] reported an increase in amplitude of the somatosensory evoked potential during pressure reversal of urethane anaesthesia and Oshimi, Shingu and Mori[45] showed increased EEG activity during halothane anaesthesia following either noxious surgical stimulation or the administration of suxamethonium.

The effect of changing sleep stage on the amplitude of the early cortical waves of the auditory evoked response has been studied in animals and man[46,47]. Whereas brainstem auditory evoked responses showed no changes with the onset of sleep, the early cortical waves decreased in amplitude and disappeared during slow wave sleep and reappeared during rapid eye movement (REM) sleep. In man, wave Pa showed no change in sleep but wave Pb (55–80 ms latency) decreased and disappeared during slow wave sleep and reappeared in REM and wakefulness.

Conclusion

These results support the hypothesis that changes in the middle latency waves of the auditory evoked responses, particularly in wave Pb, reflect depth of anaesthesia, which is the activity of the brain resulting from the balance between the arousal effects of surgical stimulation and the depressant effects of anaesthetic action. The correlation of arousal in the auditory evoked response with autonomic changes was poor and reflects the observations of Hug[1] that the latter signs are of little value in diagnosing anaesthetic depth. The auditory evoked response may also provide information about the anaesthetic concentration required to block the auditory pathway at the association area of the cortex. Thus, in addition to its promising role as a measure of depth of anaesthesia, the auditory evoked response is likely to be useful in investigating the anaesthetic action on association areas near the primary auditory cortex, and retention of and recall of high level auditory information in the nearby hippocampus. These results support the concept that the auditory evoked response reflects the balance of excitatory and inhibitory influences acting on the central nervous system and thus provides a good measure of depth of anaesthesia.

References

1. HUG, C. C. (1985) Lipid solubility, pharmacokinetics, and the EEG: are you better off today than you were four years ago? *Anesthesiology, 62,* 221–226
2. JONES, J. G. and KONIECZKO, E. (1986) Hearing and memory in anaesthetised patients. *British Medical Journal, 292,* 1291–1293
3. RUSSELL, I. F. (1986) Comparison of wakefulness with two anaesthetic regimens. Total i.v. v. balanced anaesthesia. *British Journal of Anaesthesia, 58,* 965–968
4. EDITORIAL (1979) On being aware. *British Journal of Anaesthesia, 51,* 711–712
5. MILLAR, K. and WATKINSON, N. (1982) Recognition of words presented during general anaesthesia. *Ergonomics, 26,* 585–594
6. BENNETT, H. L., DAVIS, H. S. and GIANNINI, J. A. (1985) Non-verbal response to intraoperative conversation. *British Journal of Anaesthesia, 57,* 174–179
7. BONKE, B., SCHMITZ, P. I., VERHAGE, F. and ZWAVELING, A. (1986) Clinical study of so-called unconscious perception during general anaesthesia. *British Journal of Anaesthesia, 58,* 957–964
8. JONES, J. G., HENEGHAN, C. P. H. and THORNTON, C. (1985) Functional assessment of the normal brain during general anaesthesia. In *Anaesthesia Review, 3,* edited by L. Kaufman, pp. 83–98. Edinburgh: Churchill Livingstone
9. PRIOR, P. F. (1985) EEG monitoring and evoked potentials in brain ischaemia. *British Journal of Anaesthesia, 57,* 63–81
10. LEVY, W. J., SHAPIRO, H. M., MARACHAK, G. and MEATHE, E. (1980) Automated EEG processing for intraoperative monitoring. *Anesthesiology, 53,* 223–236

11. LEVY, W. J. (1984) Intraoperative EEG patterns: implication for EEG monitoring. *Anesthesiology*, **60**, 430–434
12. RAMPIL, I. J., SASSE, F. J., SMITH, N. T., HOFF, B. H. and FLEMMING, D. C. (1980) Spectral edge frequency – a new correlate of anesthetic depth. *Anesthesiology*, **53**, 512
13. HOMER, T. D. and STANSKI, D. R. (1985) The effect of increasing age on thiopental disposition and anesthetic requirement. *Anesthesiology*, **62**, 714–724
14. ARDEN, J. R., HOLLEY, F. O. and STANSKI, D. R. (1986) Increased sensitivity to etomidate in the elderly: initial distribution versus altered brain response. *Anesthesiology*, **65**, 19–27
15. SCOTT, J. C., PONGANIS, K. U. and STANSKI, D. R. (1985) EEG quantitation of narcotic effect: the comparative pharmacodynamics of fentanyl and alfentanil. *Anesthesiology*, **62**, 224–241
16. SCHWILDEN, H., SCHUTTLER, J. and STOECKEL, H. (1985) Quantitation of the EEG and pharmacodynamic modelling of hypnotic drugs: etomidate as an example. *European Journal of Anaesthesiology*, **2**, 121–131
17. PRIOR, P. F. and MAYNARD, D. (1987) *Monitoring Cerebral Function: Long-term Monitoring of EEG and Evoked Potentials*. Amsterdam: Elsevier Science Publishers (in press)
18. CHIAPPA, K. H. and ROPPER, A. H. (1982) Evoked potentials in clinical medicine (in two parts). *New England Journal of Medicine*, **306**, 1140–1150, 1205–1211
19. DORFMAN, L. J. (1983) Sensory-evoked potentials. Clinical application in medicine. *Annual Review of Medicine*, **34**, 473–489
20. SCHMIDT, B. and BLUM, T. (1984) Retinotopic examination with magnetic encephalography. Single-channel recordings of visually evoked neuromagnetic fields. *Developments in Ophthalmology*, **9**, 46–52
21. REGAN, D. (1972) *Evoked Potentials in Psychology, Sensory Physiology and Clinical Medicine*, pp. 192–259. London: Chapman and Hall
22. HALLIDAY, A. M. (1982) The visual evoked potential in healthy subjects. In *Evoked Potentials in Clinical Testing*, edited by A. M. Halliday, *Clinical Neurology and Neurosurgery Monographs*, pp. 71–120. Edinburgh: Churchill Livingstone
23. JEWETT, D. L. and WILLISTON, J. S. (1971) Auditory-evoked far fields averaged from the scalp of humans. *Brain*, **94**, 681–696
24. KAGA, K., HINK, R. F., SHINODA, Y. and SUZUKI, J. (1980) Evidence for a primary cortical origin of middle latency auditory evoked potential in cats. *Electroencephalography and Clinical Neurophysiology*, **50**, 254–266
25. GALAMBOS, R., MAKEIG, S. and TALMACHOFF, P. J. (1981) A 40-Hz auditory potential recorded from the human scalp. *Proceedings of the National Academy of Sciences of the USA*, **78**, 2643–2647
26. THORNTON, C., CATLEY, D. M., JORDAN, C., LEHANE, J. R., ROYSTON, D. and JONES, J. G. (1983) Enflurane anaesthesia causes graded changes in the brainstem and early cortical auditory evoked response in man. *British Journal of Anaesthesia*, **55**, 479–486
27. KRISS, A., PRASHER, D. K. and PRATT, R. T. C. (1985) Brainstem and middle latency auditory EPs evoked during unilateral electroconvulsion therapy (ECT). In *Second International Evoked Potentials Symposium*, Vol. 2, edited by R. H. Nodar and C. Barber, pp. 582–588. Boston: Butterworths
28. THORNTON, C., HENEGHAN, C. P. H., NAVARATNARAJAH, M. and JONES, J. G. (1986) Selective effect of Althesin on the auditory evoked response in man. *British Journal of Anaesthesia*, **58**, 422–427
29. THORNTON, C., HENEGHAN, C. P. H., NAVARATNARAJAH, M., BATEMAN, P. E. and JONES, J. G. (1985) Effect of etomidate on the auditory evoked response in man. *British Journal of Anaesthesia*, **57**, 554–561
30. VELASCO, M., VELASCO, F., CASTENADA, R. and SANCHEZ, R. (1984) Effect of fentanyl and naloxone on humane somatic and auditory-evoked potential components. *Neuropharmacology*, **23**, 359–366
31. THORNTON, C., HENEGHAN, C. P. H., JAMES, M. F. M. and JONES, J. G. (1984) Effects of halothane or enflurane with controlled ventilation on auditory evoked potentials. *British Journal of Anaesthesia*, **56**, 315–323
32. HENEGHAN, C. P. H., THORNTON, C., NAVARATNARAJAH, M. and JONES, J. G. (1987) Effect of isoflurane on the auditory evoked response in man. *British Journal of Anaesthesia* **59**, 277–282
33. THORNTON, C., KONIECZKO, K. M., KNIGHT, A. B., KAUL, B., JONES, J. G. and WHITE, D. C. (1986) Effect of Diprivan on the auditory evoked response. *Beitrage zur Anästhesiologie und Intensivmedizin*, **16** (in press)

34. DAVIS, D. W., HAWKINS, R. A., MANS, A. M., HIBBARD, L. S. and BIEBUYCK, J. F. (1984) Regional cerebral glucose utilization during althesin anesthesia. *Anesthesiology,* **61**, 362–368

35. DAVIS, D. W., MANS, A. K., BIEBUYCK, J. F. and HAWKINS, R. A. (1986) Regional brain glucose utilization in rats during etomidate anesthesia. *Anesthesiology,* **64**, 751–757

36. YOUNG, M. L., SMITH, D. S., GREENBERG, J., REIVICH, M. and HARP, J. R. (1984) Effects of sufentanil on regional cerebral glucose utilization in rats. *Anesthesiology,* **61**, 564–568

37. MAEKAWA, T., TOMMASINO, C., SHAPIRO, H. M., KEIFER-GOODMAN, J. and KOHLENBERGER, R. W. (1986) Local cerebral blood flow and glucose utilization during isoflurane anesthesia in the rat. *Anesthesiology,* **65**, 144–151

38. ORI, C., DAM, M., PIZZOLATO, G., BATTISTIN, L. and GIRON, G. (1986) Effects of isoflurane anesthesia on local cerebral glucose utilization in the rat. *Anesthesiology,* **65**, 152–156

39. SEBEL, P. S., FLYNN, P. J. and INGRAM, D. A. (1984) Effect of nitrous oxide on visual, auditory and somatosensory evoked potentials. *British Journal of Anaesthesia,* **56**, 1403–1407

40. UHL, R. R., SQUIRES, K. C., BRUCE, D. L. and STARR, A. (1980) Effect of halothane anesthesia on the human cortical evoked response. *Anesthesiology,* **53**, 273–276

41. SEBEL, P. S., INGRAM, D. A., FLYNN, P. J., RUTHERFOORD, C. F. and ROGERS, H. (1986) Evoked potentials during isoflurane anaesthesia. *British Journal of Anaesthesia,* **58**, 580–585

42. PETERSON, D. O., DRUMMOND, J. C. and TODD, M. M. (1986) Effects of halothane, enflurane, isoflurane, and nitrous oxide on somatosensory evoked potentials in humans. *Anesthesiology,* **65**, 35–40

43. PICTON, T. W. and HILLYARD, S. A. (1974) Human auditory evoked potentials II. Effects of attention. *Electroencephalography and Clinical Neurophysiology,* **36**, 191–199

44. ANGEL, A., GRATTON, D. A., HALSEY, M. J. and WARDLEY-SMITH, B. (1980) Pressure reversal of the effect of urethane on the evoked somatosensory cortical response in the rat. *British Journal of Pharmacology,* **70**, 241–247

45. OSHIMA, E., SHINGU, K. and MORI, K. (1981) EEG activity during halothane anaesthesia in man. *British Journal of Anaesthesia,* **53**, 65–71

46. CHEN, B. M. and BUCHWALD, J. S. (1986) Midlatency auditory evoked responses: differential effects of sleep in the cat. *Electroencephalography and Clinical Neurophysiology,* **65**, 373–382

47. ERWIN, R. and BUCHWALD, J. S. (1986) Midlatency auditory evoked responses: differential effects of sleep in the human. *Electroencephalography and Clinical Neurophysiology,* **65**, 383–392

Chapter 13

Oesophageal activity and anaesthesia

J. M. Evans and D. C. White

'Then told to imagine how she would feel if suddenly informed that her boy was dead, the esophagus clamped down with lightning speed, the lumen was obliterated, and the muscle quivered.'

This is an account by Faulkner in 1940 of his observations of the effect of 'psychic factors' upon oesophageal tone as directly observed via a rigid oesophagoscope[1]. By contemporary standards the methods for both eliciting a stressful response and for observing it were far from elegant but they nevertheless demonstrated a connection between psychological stress and oesophageal activity.

The potential significance of oesophageal contractility has only recently been recognized[2]. The reason for this can probably be explained partly by the fact that the human oesophagus is unusual in the animal kingdom and partly by the fact that oesophageal physiology, and in particular physiology of the main body of the oesophagus, has not been extensively studied.

Oesophageal anatomy

The principal feature of the human oesophagus is that it is composed of striated muscle in its upper half and smooth muscle in its lower half; there is a gradual transition zone from one half to the other. The musculature of most animals, especially those traditionally used in laboratory research, is wholly striated muscle. The standard laboratory analogue for the human has been the common American opossum; more recently the baboon has also been used for studies[3].

The two halves are quite different, but the function of the two is integrated so that a peristaltic wave will pass along the length of the oesophagus giving no indication of the type of muscle providing motive power. In other respects the human oesophagus is not remarkable. An outer longitudinal muscle coat together with an inner circular coat enclose a moderately well developed *muscularis mucosae*; this in turn encloses a thin lamina propria and a mucosal lining of stratified squamous epithelium.

There is, within the wall of the oesophagus, a complex and poorly understood intramural nerve plexus. This is connected with nerve plexuses outside but adjacent to the oesophagus – the oesophageal plexus. The whole of the oesophageal nervous system is supplied with both sympathetic and parasympathetic fibres, the predominant innervation being provided by the vagus nerve which carries both afferent and efferent fibres. Central control of oesophageal motility lies in the oesophageal motility centre comprising the motor nucleus of the vagus nerve and adjacent reticular activating centre[4].

Physiology of the oesophagus

The function of the oesophagus is to convey food from the pharynx to the stomach. This function is carried out by a process referred to as *primary* peristalsis which is continuous with the oropharyngeal phase of swallowing (*Figure 13.1*). When peristalsis arises within the main body of the oesophagus without having been preceded by swallowing, and usually as a result of a fragment of a bolus of food or some other foreign body, the peristaltic response is referred to as *secondary*. In practice, it is probable that secondary peristalsis serves as a clearing up process for residual food particles in the oesophagus not cleared by the primary peristalsis. A third form of contractile activity of the oesophagus is recognized as non-peristaltic and is termed *tertiary* activity (*Figure 13.1*). There is no obvious function for this non-propulsive activity[5].

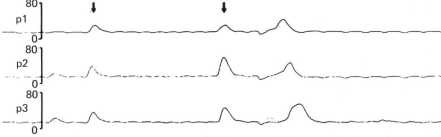

Figure 13.1 Pressure recordings from the upper (p1), middle (p2) and lower (p3) oesophagus in a conscious subject. The arrows indicate non-propulsive contractions induced by auditory stimulation. On the right is a primary peristaltic response. The non-propulsive contractions are synchronous in contrast to the primary peristaltic response on the right. (Adapted from Stacher, Schmierer and Landgraf[14])

It might appear that the oesophagus is relatively autonomous, but in fact vagal control of oesophageal function is substantial. In animals, high bilateral vagotomy produces a period of lower oesophageal paralysis[6]. Within 24–48 hours of denervation after vagotomy, local oesophageal reflexes mature, so that balloon distension of the isolated oesophagus will produce a peristaltic response[7,8]. This peristaltic response is entirely the result of local reflexes and can be observed *in vitro* in the isolated opossum oesophagus[9]. In man, however, there is strong evidence to suggest that the secondary peristaltic response (provoked lower oesophageal contraction), as observed during anaesthesia, is not this local reflex but a reflex mediated by vagal afferent and efferent connections with the brainstem oesophageal motility centre[10–12]. There is complete loss of spontaneous lower oesophageal contractions in patients with severe head injuries and clinical evidence of brainstem death. After approximately 24 hours, a low amplitude peristaltic response to balloon distension appears[13]. This form of provoked lower oesophageal contraction is characteristically of a constant value for any one subject, and not subject to the variation typically seen in anaesthetized or sedated patients. The dose–response curves for halothane upon provoked and spontaneous lower oesophageal contraction (*see below*) during anaesthesia are remarkably similar and support the proposition that the agent acts upon a single control mechanism – the oesophageal motility centre in the brainstem.

Non-propulsive activity appears not to be a function of the intact oesophagus, but to be a motor function arising in the oesophageal motility centre and facilitated from higher centres[14].

Oesophageal contractility and stress

Faulkner[1] observed oesophageal spasm endoscopically in response to psychologically disturbing questions. In a manometric study of oesophageal activity in healthy young adults, Nagler and Spiro[15] noticed that some subjects exhibited increased non-propulsive activity occasionally and, on further questioning, were able to elicit that the subjects were experiencing periods of psychological stress (e.g. induced by a threatened miscarriage in a subject's wife). Subsequently, Rubin *et al.*[16] demonstrated a relationship between periods of psychological stress during unstructured interviews and the appearance of an increase in non-propulsive activity (*Figure 13.2*). Stacher, Suter and Forster[14] induced non-propulsive

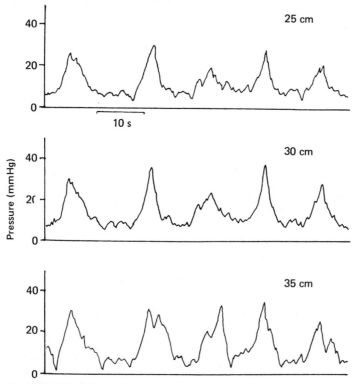

Figure 13.2 Pressure recordings from the upper, middle and lower thirds of the oesophagus. The recordings clearly demonstrate much non-propulsive activity in a conscious subject – typically associated with enhanced emotional responses. (Adapted from Rubin *et al.*[16])

contractions in the oesophagus by acoustic stimulation (*see Figure 13.1*); a possible explanation for this consistent response was not immediately clear. It may be a 'startle' response, but the fact that it could be obtained repetitively suggested that this was unlikely; a possible reflex defensive response may provide an explanation.

The above work indicates a clear relationship between psychological stress, or stimulation, and non-propulsive oesophageal activity. The commonly recognized 'lump in the throat' experienced during moments of psychological distress may be an intense non-propulsive contraction of the whole of the body of the oesophagus, including the cricopharyngeal muscles.

Oesophageal pharmacology

A distinction has to be drawn between the main body of the oesophagus and the lower oesophageal sphincter. There is a significant pharmacological difference between these two structures: the lower oesophageal sphincter appear to be very much more susceptible to drug effects than does the main body of the oesophagus[17].

Skeletal muscle relaxants suppress motility of the upper half of the oesophagus. Despite full skeletal muscle paralysis, lower oesophageal motility remains preserved[2,18]. Smooth muscle relaxants, such as sodium nitroprusside in high therapeutic doses, produce complete paralysis of the lower half of the oesophagus. It is probable that other smooth muscle relaxants have the same effects. A reduction in spontaneous contraction rate of 50% has been observed during hypothermia (28 °C) for cardiac surgery (D. Thomas, personal communication).

The predominant synaptic mechanism involved in the control of oesophageal contractility is cholinergic, and thus the anticholinergic drugs are capable of producing a dose-dependent depression of activity. Some interference can be identified in patients given intramuscular atropine 1 hour pre-operatively in routine doses; substantial interference is produced by intravenous atropine[18]. Cholinergic agents increase oesophageal activity[15].

Very few α- and β-adrenergic receptors are present in the lower oesophagus. Those that are present are mostly associated with blood vessels, and oesophageal activity has been recorded in patients who were receiving therapeutic doses of α- and β-antagonists[4]. It would be expected that metoclopramide would increase lower oesophageal activity, but this effect has not been observed following intravenous increments of 10 mg in anaesthetized subjects.

Lower oesophageal contractility and anaesthesia

The measurement of lower oesophageal contractility, as a means of eliciting evidence of light anaesthesia, has been largely confined to intubated, paralysed and ventilated patients.

Lower oesophageal contractility is not usually recorded in the intubated patient breathing spontaneously, because that dose of anaesthetic which suppresses the response to a tracheal tube is usually sufficient to suppress oesophageal contractility.

The background signal

The intrinsic tone of the oesophagus during anaesthesia is minimal, only about 1 or 2 mmHg. The effect of therapeutic doses of anaesthetic agents on the resting tone of the lower oesophagus is small[17]. *Figure 13.3* shows a pressure recording obtained from a balloon-tipped catheter from the lower oesophagus (35 cm from the lips) in a paralysed, ventilated and anaesthetized patient. There is a regular pressure cycle of approximately 10 mmHg in amplitude, synchronous with positive pressure ventilation of the lungs; this is transmitted pressure from within the intrathoracic cavity. A more detailed examination of the recording at higher speeds and greater amplitude shows a cardiac impulse superimposed upon the respiratory cycle. It is thus possible to record pulmonary and cardiac artefacts in the lower oesophagus, but the amplitudes of these seldom exceed 10 or 15 mmHg.

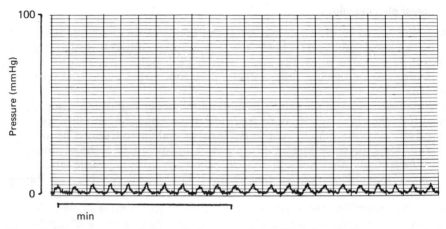

Figure 13.3 A pressure recording from the lower oesophagus (35 cm from lips) in an anaesthetized, paralysed, ventilated patient. Transmitted positive pressure ventilation artefacts are obvious and small cardiac artefacts can also be discerned

Spontaneous lower oesophageal contractions

Spontaneous contractions of the lower oesophagus typical of those seen during light anaesthesia are shown in *Figure 13.4*. If additional pressure measurements are made in the lower, middle and upper third of the oesophagus (*Figure 13.5*), it is apparent that the contractions of the lower oesophagus are synchronous with simultaneous contractions in the middle and upper third. The contraction is therefore not peristaltic but non-propulsive, similar to those observed in conscious subjects during periods of psychological stress (*see Figure 13.2*). It has been shown (*see below*) that, within therapeutic doses, the anaesthetic agents have no effect upon the *amplitude* of spontaneous lower oesophageal contractions but have a marked effect upon their *rate*.

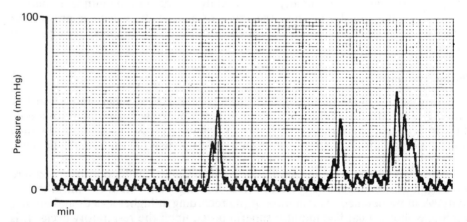

Figure 13.4 Spontaneous lower oesophageal contractions in an anaesthetized, paralysed, ventilated patient. These develop during lightening anaesthesia and have an amplitude very much greater than the baseline signal. (Adapted from Evans, Davies and Wise[2])

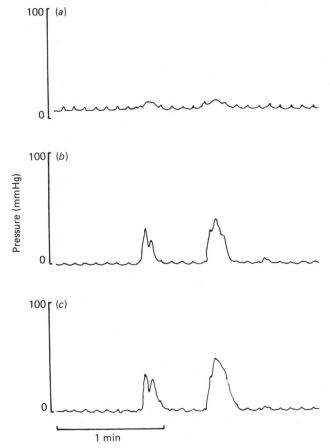

Figure 13.5 Pressure recordings from the (*a*) upper, (*b*) middle and (*c*) lower oesophagus in an anaesthetized, paralysed, ventilated patient. Paralysis of the skeletal muscle of the upper oesophagus almost completely suppresses upper oesophageal activity. The contractions are not peristaltic, but synchronous non-propulsive contractions similar to those seen in *Figures 13.1* and *13.2*. (Adapted from Evans, Davies and Wise[2])

The similarity of recordings of spontaneous lower oesophageal contractions during anaesthesia and non-propulsive contractions in conscious subjects, and the association of these contractions with light anaesthesia, would suggest that their appearance during anaesthesia is an indication that the patient is developing a stress response similar to that induced by psychological or acoustic stimulation in conscious subjects. It is presumed that it is a motor response of the vagal motor nuclei facilitated by higher centres. The amplitude of spontaneous contractions is typically between 30 and 40 mmHg, but in some patients it may exceed 100 mmHg. The amplitude may be depressed by drugs which interfere with oesophageal activity. However, the amplitude of the response does not appear to be very relevant; it is the frequency that is significant and, providing spontaneous lower oesophageal contractions can be identified and their rate measured, then the observation will be of value.

Provoked lower oesophageal contractility

In a conscious subject, the inflation of a balloon in the oesophagus will produce a secondary peristaltic response. The same effect can be observed during anaesthesia. In the lightly anaesthetized patient, balloon distension of the oesophagus can induce a secondary peristaltic response.

The probe shown in *Figure 13.6* has two balloons. The smaller distal balloon is liquid filled and coupled to an external pressure transducer. The proximal balloon is air filled and can be inflated to a diameter of 15 mm. The brief inflation of this

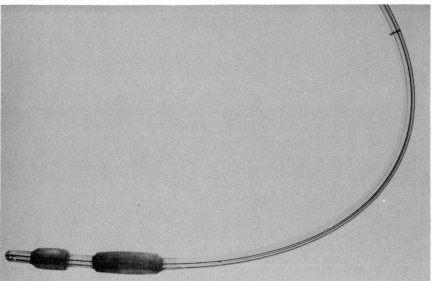

Figure 13.6 An oesophageal probe with a small distal pressure measuring balloon (coupled to an external pressure transducer) and a larger proximal balloon used both as an oesophageal stethoscope and, on inflation, to produce a secondary peristaltic response in the oesophagus

proximal balloon will provoke a secondary peristaltic response, which will be seen by the pressure-sensing balloon as a passing peristaltic wave, usually identical in appearance to a non-propulsive contraction (*Figure 13.7*). During deep anaesthesia, a provoked contraction is not obtained; as anaesthesia lightens, the provoked contraction appears with increasing amplitude as the supply of anaesthetic is decreased. Thus, in contrast to spontaneous contractions, the *amplitude* of the provoked response is related to the degree of anaesthesia.

The neurophysiological mechanism of provoked lower oesophageal contractility is not entirely clear. There is considerable similarity between primary and secondary peristaltic responses[10] in conscious subjects and, in anaesthetized patients, the dose–effect curves for halothane on spontaneous contraction rate and on provoked contraction amplitude[19] are very similar. This suggests that there is a common mechanism for the responses and favours the proposition that the provoked response involves afferent and efferent connections to the brainstem motor nucleus. It is not clear, however, whether the secondary peristaltic response is the result of a sequential firing of neurones in the brainstem nucleus or whether the brainstem nucleus initiates a peristaltic response which is controlled by oesophageal and para-oesophageal reflexes[20].

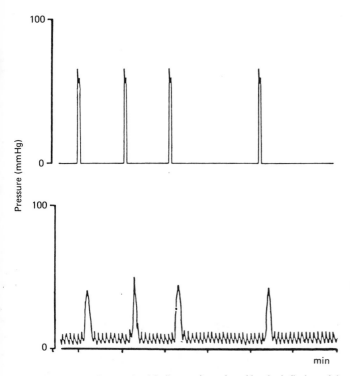

Figure 13.7 Secondary peristalsis (bottom) produced by the inflation of the provoking balloon (top) on the probe in an anaesthetized patient. (Adapted from Evans, Davies and Wise[2])

Lower oesophageal contractility and intravenous anaesthetics

Althesin

The effect of Althesin (alphaxalone–alphadalone) has been studied in paralysed patients ventilated with 50% nitrous oxide[21]. The adequacy of anaesthesia was judged by clinical means and increments of intravenous Althesin were given on the basis of clinical signs (blood pressure, heart rate, sweating, lacrimation and pupil size) while lower oesophageal contractility was recorded blind to the anaesthetist. An analysis of the recordings, before and after the decision to inject another increment of Althesin, is shown in *Figures 13.8* and *13.9*. As anaesthesia lightened, the spontaneous contraction rate increased to almost 4 contractions/min and decreased, after the administration of Althesin, to a low of a little under 1 contraction/min. The depression was maximal at about 3 minutes after administration. In contrast, Althesin had no effect upon the amplitude of spontaneous contractions. This suggests that the spontaneous contraction response is an 'all or none' response and, once triggered, proceeds autonomously to completion. The effect of Althesin upon provoked contractility was not investigated in this study.

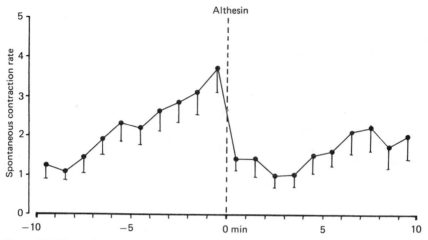

Figure 13.8 Change in spontaneous lower oesophageal contraction rate before and after administration of Althesin (mean, s.e.). (Adapted from Evans, Davies and Wise[21])

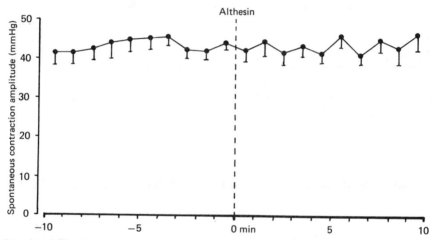

Figure 13.9 Changes in spontaneous lower oesophageal contraction mean amplitude before and after administration of Althesin (mean, s.e.). Althesin, in contrast to spontaneous contraction rate, had no effect upon mean spontaneous contraction amplitude

Methohexitone

The effect of methohexitone upon lower oesophageal contractility has been studied by Brady and Clarke[22]. Anaesthesia was maintained by an infusion of methohexitone which was varied so as to produce a range of 'depths' of anaesthesia. Deep anaesthesia was associated with a diminished spontaneous contraction rate and provoked contraction amplitude and light anaesthesia with an increase in spontaneous contraction rate and provoked contraction amplitude before there was clinical evidence. Acceptable clinical anaesthesia was, typically, associated with a spontaneous contraction rate of 0.5–1 contraction/min and provoked amplitude of around 20 mmHg.

Intravenous analgesics

Both morphine and fentanyl, given as a supplement to nitrous oxide anaesthesia, produce a depression of spontaneous contraction rate and provoked contraction amplitude. The degree and duration of suppression by any given dose is very variable and probably reflects their variable anaesthetic properties.

The effect of an increment of 5 mg of morphine is shown in *Figure 13.10*. Lower oesophageal contractility returned to pre-increment activity after approximately 30 minutes.

Fentanyl has a comparable action; fentanyl requirements and lower oesophageal contractility are described below in connection with closed-loop control of anaesthesia.

Measurements of lower oesophageal contractility have been used to monitor and control the sedation of paralysed, ventilated patients receiving intensive care. The effect of an infusion of midazolam and morphine has been monitored by the lower oesophageal contractility response so that inappropriate sedation of the patients could be avoided[13].

Propofol

Initial pilot investigation indicates that propofol has an effect comparable to Althesin, but a systematic study has not yet been completed.

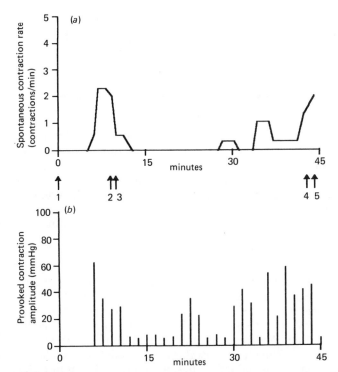

Figure 13.10 Spontaneous (*a*) and provoked (*b*) contractions during anaesthesia.
(1) Induction and intubation: thiopentone 500 mg, atracurium 35 mg and morphine 2.5 mg. Maintenance: O_2, 70% N_2O, intermittent positive pressure ventilation. (2) Skin incision; (3) morphine 5 mg; (4) atropine/neostigmine; (5) extubation

Lower oesophageal contractility and inhalational anaesthetics

Halothane

Preliminary investigation of the effect of halothane upon spontaneous and provoked contractions shows a progressive dose reduction in the rate of spontaneous contractions and the amplitude of provoked contractions. At 2.0 MAC (where MAC = minimum alveolar concentration at which 50% subjects react to a specified stimulus) virtually complete suppression of both indices was obtained (*Figure 13.11*). At 1.0 MAC, the spontaneous contraction rate was 0.6 contraction/min while the provoked contractility was 15 mmHg^2. A more extensive investigation of the effect of halothane confirms this relationship[19].

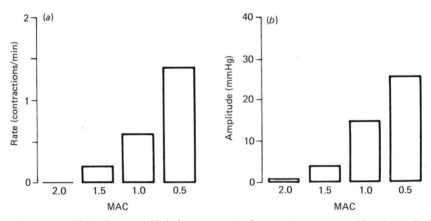

Figure 13.11 Effect of a range of halothane concentrations upon spontaneous (*a*) and provoked (*b*) lower oesophageal contractility measured in one subject. (Adapted from Evans, Davies and Wise[2])

Changes in spontaneous contraction rate and provoked contractility amplitude, recorded during a preliminary investigation of the affect of halothane anaesthesia upon lower oesophageal contractility, are shown in *Figure 13.12*. The changes in these are correlated with a clinical score (PRST score, *see* Chapter 4) which ranges in value from 0 to 8 – the useful range of this in practice is 0 to 4, 0 correlating with deep anaesthesia, and 4 with light anaesthesia. In both instances, light anaesthesia was associated with an increase in the two lower oesophageal contractility indices.

Isoflurane

Isoflurane, added to 66% nitrous oxide, at an end-expired concentration greater than 0.8% produced suppression of lower oesophageal contractility in 90% of patients. At end-expired concentrations of less than 0.4%, 90% of patients showed lower oesophageal contractility. In this study of 30 patients, three showed no contractions at any time and nine appeared clinically 'light' despite the absence of lower oesophageal contractility[23]. The effect of isoflurane upon lower oesophageal contractility during anaesthesia for an abdominal hysterectomy is shown in *Figure 13.13*. In an investigation of the effect of graded concentrations of isoflurane, a similar dose–response curve to that for halothane has been obtained (J. M. Calkins, personal communication).

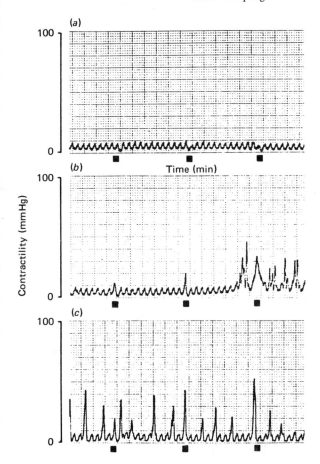

Figure 13.12 Recordings of lower oesophageal contractility and associated PRST scores and concentration of halothane; the square markers indicate provocation. (*a*) MAC = 1.5; PRST = 1; maximum provoked contraction = 1 mmHg; spontaneous contraction rate = 0; (*b*) MAC = 1.0; PRST = 2, maximum provoked contraction = 14 mmHg; spontaneous contraction rate = 0.32 contraction/min; (*c*) MAC = 0.5; PRST = 3; maximum provoked contraction = 31 mmHg; spontaneous contraction rate = 0.44/min

Enflurane

No systematic study of enflurane has been performed, but it behaves rather like halothane and isoflurane. The changes in lower oesophageal contractility during a nitrous oxide/enflurane anaesthesia are shown in *Figure 13.14*.

Lower oesophageal contractility and control of anaesthesia

A preliminary investigation of the potential value of using lower oesophageal contractility to control anaesthetic supply has been undertaken[24,25]. A simple closed-loop control system was developed based only on spontaneous contractions.

124

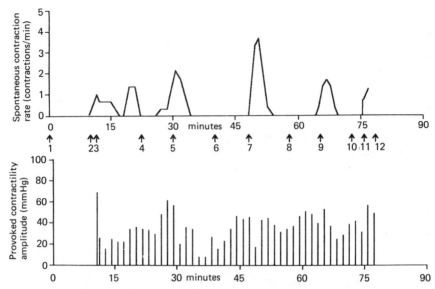

Figure 13.13 Isoflurane and lower oesophageal contractility.
(1) Induction and intubation: thiopentone 350 mg; pancuronium 7 mg; fentanyl 100 μg. Maintenance: intermittent positive pressure ventilation, O_2, 70% N_2O, 1% isoflurane. (2) Isoflurane increased to 1.5%; (3) skin incision; (4) isoflurane increased to 4.0%; (5) isoflurane decreased to 2.0%; (6) isoflurane decreased to 0.0%; (7) isoflurane increased to 1.5%; (8) isoflurane decreased to 0.0%; (9) isoflurane increased to 1.0%; (10) isoflurane decreased to 0.0%; (11) atropine/neostigmine; (12) extubated

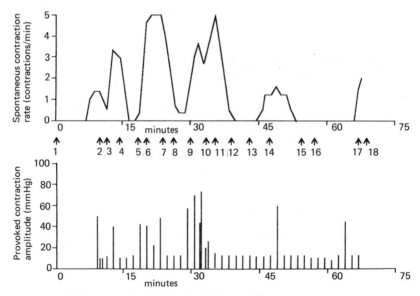

Figure 13.14 Enflurane and lower oesophageal contractility.
(1) Induction and intubation: thiopentone 350 mg; pancuronium 7 mg; fentanyl 100 μg. Maintenance: O_2, 70% N_2O, 1.5% enflurane, intermittent positive pressure ventilation. (2) Enflurane increased to 4%; (3) skin incision; (4) enflurane reduced to 2%; (5) enflurane reduced to 1%; (6) enflurane increased to 2%; (7) enflurane increased to 4%; (8) enflurane reduced to 2%; (9) enflurane increased to 4%; (10) enflurane reduced to 3%; (11) fentanyl 100 μg; (12) enflurane reduced to 2%; (13) enflurane reduced to 1%; (14) enflurane increased to 1.5%; (15) enflurane reduced to 0.5%; (16) enflurane off; (17) atropine/neostigmine; (18) extubated

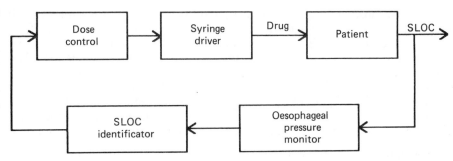

Figure 13.15 Schematic diagram of lower oesophageal contractility closed-loop control system. Spontaneous contraction (SLOC) was monitored by an oesophageal pressure monitor – spontaneous contraction greater than 15 mmHg was identified and each event over threshold triggered a preset intravenous dose of drug to be delivered by the syringe driver

For every spontaneous contraction in excess of a preset threshold (15 mmHg), an increment of drug was supplied to the patient (*Figure 13.15*). Induction of anaesthesia was with thiopentone, fentanyl 1 µg and pancuronium; then the patients' lungs were ventilated with 70% nitrous oxide. Thereafter, the supply of additional fentanyl was determined by spontaneous contraction activity. One spontaneous contraction resulted in the supplemental administration of 5 µg/70 kg. The uptake of fentanyl in five subjects is shown in *Figure 13.16.*

A number of features emerge from this. First, the initial loading dose of fentanyl has a very variable effect; in some patients (patient A), the demand for fentanyl commences almost immediately the closed-loop system is connected (at 10

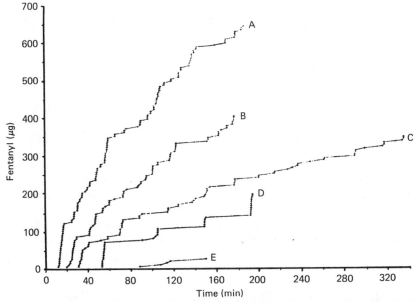

Figure 13.16 Infusion of fentanyl in five patients controlled by spontaneous contraction activity using the closed-loop control system. Demand commenced almost immediately in patient A and remained high thereafter. In patient E, demand did not commence for 90 minutes and thereafter was very low. In patient D oscillation of the control system is apparent

minutes), while in others the effect of the initial loading dose persists for up to 90 minutes (patient E). In those patients in whom the loading dose has the least effect, the demand rate thereafter is very high; in contrast, in those patients in whom the loading has the most prolonged effect, the demand rate thereafter is low. The control system was a simple 'bang-bang' system which is very inclined to oscillate. Patient D exhibits this effect with bursts of feedback at intervals of approximately 50 minutes. The general pattern of uptake has a characteristic form, with an initial exponential phase and a dominant linear phase towards the end of the procedure. The form of the equation for the line which is the best fit to the results is as follows:

$$\text{Fentanyl uptake} = -a + bt + c \log t$$

where a, b and c are constants and t = time.

The ratio of demand for the five subjects was 100:1 after 100 minutes of anaesthesia. All patients recovered rapidly after anaesthesia, and the average time to opening eyes and obeying commands after atropine and neostigmine and stopping fentanyl and nitrous oxide, was 5.3 minutes.

This suggests that lower oesophageal contractility is sensitive to individual demand for anaesthetic requirement. Furthermore, the prompt recovery of the patients despite considerable variation in dosage suggests that this is an appropriate indicator of requirement. Finally, the nature of uptake is consistent with the decay of the initial loading dose and the attempts of the closed-loop control system to maintain a steady state. At no time were the patients deemed clinically to be either too light or too deep; no patient had any recall of intra-operative events.

Limitations of lower oesophageal contractility monitoring

The outline of oesophageal physiology and pharmacology indicates clearly some of the potential limitations of lower oesophageal contractility in clinical practice. Pharmacological interference will be produced by, and largely confined to, drugs with smooth muscle relaxant or anticholinergic effects; although lower oesophageal contractility may not be entirely normal, the measurement may still be of value if the rate of spontaneous contractions can be identified. Significant local oesophageal disease, such as achalasia or scleroderma, will similarly interfere. Diseases of the autonomic nervous system have the potential for altering autonomic reflexes and diabetic autonomic neuropathy warrants investigation in this respect.

A reduction in lower oesophageal sphincter tone can be observed in pregnancy, although no obvious difference in lower oesophageal activity was found in a pilot study of lower oesophageal contractility, and general anaesthesia for caesarean section[26].

Surgery in the vicinity of the pharynx, larynx or oesophagus may provide additional mechanical stimulation of the system and may cause an increase in activity.

Lower oesophageal contractility and awareness

It remains to be seen whether monitoring lower oesophageal contractility will assist in the prevention of awareness. There is certainly a correlation between anaesthetic depth and lower oesophageal contractility, which should provide the anaesthetist with some additional guidance on the adequacy of anaesthesia. The observations of increasing non-propulsive activity (spontaneous contractions) in conscious patients, subject to relatively modest psychological stress, leads us to believe that any significant level of comparable stress during inadequate anaesthesia would certainly be reflected in an increase in lower oesophageal contractility activity. It is thus possible that awareness accompanied by distress may be manifest by an increase in lower oesophageal contractility. Equally, it is possible that awareness unaccompanied by distress in a patient who is pain free may not generate a marked increase in lower oesophageal contractility.

References

1. FAULKNER, W. B. (1940) Objective esophageal changes due to psychic factors. Esophagoscopic study with a report of 13 cases. *American Journal of Medical Science*, **200**, 796–803
2. EVANS, J. M., DAVIES, W. L. and WISE, C. C. (1984) Lower oesophageal contractility: a new monitor of anaesthesia. *Lancet*, **i**, 1151–1154
3. BROWN, F. C., GIDEON, R. M., VOELKER, F. A. and CASTELL, D. D. (1978) Muscle function and structure of the esophagus of the baboon (*Papio anubis*). *American Journal of Veterinary Research*, **39**, 1209–1211
4. CHRISTENSEN, J. (1978) The innervation and motility of the esophagus. *Frontiers of Gastrointestinal Research*, **3**, 18–32
5. INGELFINGER, F. J. (1958) Esophageal motility. *Physiological Reviews*, **38**, 533–584
6. HIGGS, B. and ELLIS, F. H. (1965) The effect of bilateral supranodosal vagotomy on canine esophageal function. *Surgery*, **58**, 828–834
7. CANNON, W. B. (1907) Esophageal peristalsis after bilateral vagotomy. *American Journal of Physiology*, **19**, 436–444
8. REYNOLDS, R. P. E., EL-SHARKAWY, T. Y. and DIAMANT, N. E. (1985) Oesophageal peristalsis in the cat: the role of central innervation assessed by transient vagal blockade. *Canadian Journal of Physiology and Pharmacology*, **63**, 122–130
9. CHRISTENSEN, J. and LUND, G. F. (1969) Esophageal responses to distension and electrical stimulation. *Journal of Clinical Investigation*, **48**, 408–419
10. SIEGEL, C. I. and HENDRIX, T. R. (1961) Evidence for the central mediation of secondary peristalsis in the esophagus. *Bulletin of the Johns Hopkins Hospital*, **108**, 297–307
11. ENZMANN, D. R., HARELL, G. S. and ZBORALSKE, F. F. (1977) Upper esophageal responses to intraluminal distension in man. *Gastroenterology*, **72**, 1292–1298
12. BURGESS, J. N., SCHLEGEL, J. F. and ELLIS, F. H. (1972) The effect of denervation on feline esophageal function and morphology. *Journal of Surgical Research*, **12**, 24–33
13. SINCLAIR, M. E., SUTER, P. M. and FORSTER, A. (1986) Monitoring lower oesophageal activity in the ITU. *Proceedings of 3rd European Congress of Intensive Care*, Hamburg, June 1986
14. STACHER, G., SCHMIERER, G. and LANDGRAF, M. (1979) Tertiary esophageal contractions evoked by acoustical stimuli. *Gastroenterology*, **77**, 49–54
15. NAGLER, R. and SPIRO, H. M. (1961) Serial esophageal motility studies in asymptomatic young subjects. *Gastroenterology*, **41**, 371–379
16. RUBIN, J., NAGLER, R., SPIRO, H. M. and PILOT, M. L. (1986) Measuring the effect of emotions on esophageal motility. *Psychosomatic Medicine*, **24**, 170–176
17. SEHHATI, G., FREY, R. and STAR, E. G. (1980) The action of inhalation anesthetics upon the lower esophageal sphincter. *Acta Anaesthesiologica Belgica*, **2**, 91–98
18. KANTROWITZ, P. A., SIEGEL, C. I., STRONG, M. J. and HENDRIX, T. R. (1970) Response of the human oesophagus to *d*-tubocurarine and atropine. *Gut*, **11**, 47–50
19. EVANS, J. M. (1985) Lower oesophageal contractility (LOC) during halothane anaesthesia. *British Journal of Anaesthesia*, **57**, 815P–816P
20. MUKHOPADHYAY, A. K. and WEISBRODT, N. W. (1975) Neural organization of esophageal peristalsis: role of vagus nerve. *Gastroenterology*, **68**, 444–447

21. EVANS, J. M., DAVIES, W. L. and WISE, C. C. (1985) Effect of Althesin upon spontaneous lower oesophageal contractility (SLOC) in man. *British Journal of Anaesthesia,* **57**, 340P
22. BRADY, M. M. and CLARKE, R. S. J. (1985) Assessing the depth of anaesthesia using an oesophageal contractility monitor. *Irish Journal of Medical Science,* **154**, 333
23. COX, P. N. and WHITE, D. C. (1986) Do oesophageal contractions measure 'depth' of anaesthesia? *British Journal of Anaesthesia,* **58**, 131P–132P
24. EVANS, J. M., DAVIES, W. L., FRASER, A. and WISE, C. C. (1981) Servo-controlled intravenous anaesthesia. *Proceedings of Control Techniques in Anaesthesia and Drug Administration.* Institute of Measurement and Control, London, May 1981
25. EVANS, J. M., FRASER, A., WISE, C. C. and DAVIES, W. L. (1983) Computer controlled anesthesia. In *Computing in Anesthesia and Intensive Care,* edited by O. Prakash, pp. 279–291. Boston: Martinus Nijhoff
26. THOMAS, D. and EVANS, J. M. (1985) 'Depth of anesthesia' monitoring during general anesthesia for caesarean section. *Proceedings of Society for Obstetric Anesthesia and Perinatology,* Washington, May 1985

Chapter 14

A hypothetical application of PET to determine the concentration of anaesthetic at the site of action

W. W. Mapleson

Measurements of depth of anaesthesia are necessarily imprecise, because there can probably never be a strict quantitative scale of measurement. However, in principle, it should be possible to measure the concentration of anaesthetic at the site of action, and this could provide a relatively precise datum to which different measures of depth of anaesthesia could be referenced. In order to achieve this, it is necessary, not only to be able to measure the concentration at some site, presumably in the brain, but also to determine the anatomical location of that site. It seems possible that, after considerable refinement, positive emission tomography (PET) scanning might make both these determinations possible.

The principle of the method is as follows. *Figure 14.1* shows curves which indicate how, according to a simplified form of established pharmacokinetic theory[1], the partial pressure, or tension, of an inhaled anaesthetic increases with time at the site of action. The three curves correspond to the administration of the anaesthetic at three different constant inspired tensions, in three separate hypothetical experiments in one subject. The horizontal line represents the tension required at the site for loss of consciousness (or any well-defined level of unconsciousness). This is assumed to be the same in all three experiments. The three intersections (○) indicate the times at which loss of consciousness occurs in the three experiments. In *Figure 14.2*, three further curves (broken lines) have been added to indicate the rise in tension at another site, with a lesser perfusion, in the same three experiments. At this other site, the tensions at the moment of loss of consciousness, indicated by the intersections (×), are different in the three experiments.

The principle of the method was used in a study of the induction of anaesthesia with nitrous oxide[2,3]. Two volunteers were anaesthetized with various inhaled tensions, including hyperbaric tensions, on different occasions. Loss of consciousness was indicated by the subject ceasing to press a button in response to pre-recorded sequential spoken numbers, broadcast from a tape recorder at regular, 3-second intervals. A computer model of the distribution of nitrous oxide in the body was developed and shown to predict measured values of accumulated uptake of nitrous oxide and of the end-tidal concentration of nitrous oxide. The model was then used to compute, for each experiment, the tension at the moment of loss of consciousness in various parts of the brain defined, not anatomically, but in terms of their perfusion. By interpolation between the results for the different perfusions, a perfusion was found which came nearest to giving the same computed

Tension

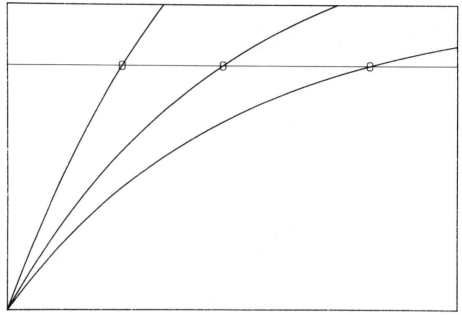

Time

Figure 14.1 Theoretical curves for the increase in the tension of an inhaled anaesthetic at the site of action for three hypothetical experiments, conducted with three different constant inhaled tensions. The horizontal line indicates the tension required for loss of consciousness and the three intersections (O) indicate the theoretical times of loss of consciousness. (Each curve is plotted as a single-exponential approach to its asymptote; in reality the approaches would be multi-exponential, but the principle would be unaltered)

tension in all experiments. As a result, the site of action was defined as one having a perfusion of the order of 1–3 ml/min per ml of tissue.

To utilize the principle with PET scanning, it would be necessary to take a 'snapshot' of the brain at the moment of loss of consciousness in each experiment, and look for that part of the brain which had the same concentration of anaesthetic in all experiments. Thus, with this approach, the site of action would be determined *anatomically*. Once this was achieved, the concentration at the site of action could be monitored in further subjects, and changes related to changes in other estimates of levels of consciousness.

This approach may never be practicable because of limitations of PET scanning. Thus, the theoretical limit to resolution is 2.5–3 mm. There will be interference from changing activity in the blood flowing through the site of action. A 'snapshot' takes of the order of 1 min, which is the whole of the 'time-to-no-response' in many of the nitrous oxide experiments. There may not be a single site of action and, even if there is, the method will not discriminate against a site with the same perfusion as that of the site of action.

However, perhaps some other technique will be developed which will overcome at least some of these difficulties. The principle could already be used to give a

Tension

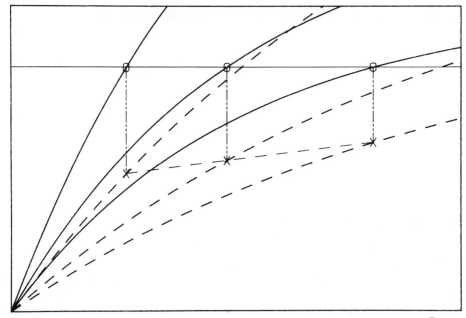

Time

Figure 14.2 As for *Figure 14.1* but with additional curves (broken lines) for another site, with a lesser perfusion. Note that, at the times of loss of consciousness, the tension at this other site is different in the three hypothetical experiments

more precise estimate of the *perfusion* of the site of action: it would be necessary to repeat the nitrous oxide experiments (which were not designed for this purpose) with some lower inspired tensions included in the series.

References

1. MAPLESON, W. W. (1973) Circulation-time models of the uptake of inhaled anaesthetics and data for quantifying them. *British Journal of Anaesthesia,* **45**, 319–334
2. MAPLESON, W. W., SMITH, W. D. A., SIEBOLD, K., HARGREAVES, M. D. and CLARKE, G. M. (1974) Nitrous oxide anaesthesia induced at atmospheric and hyperbaric pressures. Part II: Comparison of measured and theoretical pharmacokinetic data. *British Journal of Anaesthesia,* **46**, 13–28
3. SMITH, W. D. A., MAPLESON, W. W., SIEBOLD, K., HARGREAVES, M. D. and CLARKE, G. M. (1974) Nitrous oxide anaesthesia induced at atmospheric and hyperbaric pressures. Part I: Measured pharmacokinetic and EEG data. *British Journal of Anaesthesia,* **46**, 3–12

Chapter 15

Learning and memory in anaesthesia

H. L. Bennett

Anaesthetists, who usually use precise terms and make very fine distinctions between modes of pharmaceutical action, have crude and inaccurate beliefs about the activity of higher functions such as sensation, perception, memory, consciousness, and awareness. It is common, for example, for anaesthetists to say that patients 'go to sleep' when anaesthesia is induced, or that they are 'put out'. The patients' skeletal muscles are unresponsive and they have amnesia after the anaesthetic, but this view neglects a wide range of responsiveness. Lack of movement serves as one criterion for anaesthesia. Another function of the central nervous system, the perceptual or input side, is apparently ignored. Yet this input side must be differentiated from the output side, both conceptually and neurophysiologically. A major point of this chapter will be that registration of sensory events, especially auditory registrations, can occur during adequate anaesthesia with post-anaesthetic consequences, yet neither has the patient been inadequately anaesthetized nor has he a conscious memory of the event.

The input side must be examined electrophysiologically to observe that sensory registration continues deep into the central nervous system virtually unaltered, especially for auditory events. The raw EEG may be profoundly changed by anaesthetics, temperature, and biochemical events, but the response at the cortex to auditory signals simply does not change, or if it changes, it changes minimally. A flat EEG induced by barbiturates still shows an averaged evoked response to an auditory signal. Rats can be conditioned, in a pavlovian manner, under anaesthesia[1]. Studies with auditory evoked potentials support this conclusion: using signal averaging, auditory sounds are preserved under all levels of ordinary clinical anaesthesia. Auditory functioning should, therefore, be considered functionally intact.

It is one thing to argue that signals are undoubtedly arriving at the auditory cortex, but quite another to state that they can have any consequence. The signals may, for example, simply have no lasting impression; they may not activate knowledge structures.

There are well-controlled studies which have examined this matter. If the studies have examined the ability of the person to retrieve consciously or to recall the information presented during anaesthesia, then there is a dense amnesia, and performance is at chance levels. If, on the other hand, the investigators understand and anticipate the conscious amnesia and design their study to examine memory systems which do not rely upon conscious memory, then language messages presented during adequate general anaesthesia have been shown not only to register and remain but also to affect, sometimes profoundly, the post-operative behaviour and the emotional states of patients.]

An implicit assumption about the anaesthetized patient is that what we know as mental activity has ceased entirely and we are witness to a lump of perfused tissue, a functionally decorticated mass of in-flows and out-flows. The 'person' has disappeared. These processes, believed to be mental, are probably biological. The biological systems may remain functional, but normal consciousness is ablated during adequate anaesthesia. Thus, listening, as conscious perception, does not occur but hearing as the registration of auditory information may continue as an automatic neurological process.

Memory retrieval: case reports

The history of anecdotal case reports in the literature shows that, often, conscious memory was not apparent until some significant time after surgery. The report is invariably of a significant rather than a trivial incident[2].

The most common disparaging remark made in the operating room about the anesthetized patient is probably in reference to weight[3-5]. The fact that several days elapse before the patients recall the insults is consistent with the experimental results reviewed later. Insulting remarks by the surgeon and then post-operative effects (or not) on affect and vegetative processes are described elsewhere[5-9].

The case report literature helps inform about the issues of perception and memory for intra-operative events, but nearly all adequate anaesthetics produce amnesia such that patients are satisfied that they cannot recall the events of surgery. When unexpected recall occurs, after apparently adequate anaesthesia, it is for meaningful events. Responsiveness and high level communication with patients can take place during some light anaesthetics yet there is usually conscious amnesia following surgery.

Memory retrieval: experimental studies

A review by Trustman, Dubovsky, and Titley was the first rigorous one to make sense of the claims relevant to intra-operative perception and memory[10]. Other reviewers make similar points[11,12]. There are several experimental studies[3,4,9,13-17] which have used different methods to unravel this problem. Memory and learning can be assessed by the use of homophones, spelling improvements, or general recognition tests, and most workers have concluded that there is evidence of auditory input affecting memory, although conscious efforts subsequently were usually ineffective in bringing the new information to light.

Studies by Adam[18] support the proposition that assessment of learning during anaesthesia should be conducted later rather than sooner after exposure to the anaesthetics. Subanaesthetic concentrations of different gaseous anaesthetics were administered to human volunteers. Through a learn–test–retest design, Adam estimated the savings of verbal and non-verbal material over time following recovery from the anaesthetics. Amnesia was typically dense immediately following subanaesthetic learning, but recovery of material increased over time to the end of the 2-week test period. Thus, rather than a deficit of memory formation, Adam's results indicate a 'permanent inaccessibility of traces'. The memory exists, but conscious memory strategies were not able to access the information.

All of the above studies used words, or lists of paired words, that have no relevance to the concerns of the surgical patients.

The nervous system has, however, a greater response for evaluative, survival-type messages than for word lists. Conversation in the operating room resumed after the word lists were no longer read and perceptual mechanisms continued although the experiment was over. Much more pertinent things are said during operations, which is an incredibly personal and vulnerable time, and are such that perceptual systems may respond in more elaborate ways to potent stimuli than to word lists.

Memory assessed non-verbally

The fact that a few patients recall conversations, especially if highly motivated, signifies the potential for information to be assimilated into the central nervous system. Might this information affect the status of the body and psychological well-being, even though the information never entered consciousness? This is the intent of research which recognizes the dense *conscious* post-operative amnesia, yet asks if high level stimulus registration may continue during anaesthesia with post-operative results. This approach does not depend on verbal retrieval as the sole criterion to assess whether stimulus acquisition has happened.

One easily utilized and well-established way of activating response tendencies by verbal means is through the use of suggestion. Suggestions act as procedural instructions which, when combined with a delay in time until their activation or retrieval, qualify as memories. Suggestions may act by engaging early pre-attentive levels of the knowledge base because little attentional effort is involved. Thus, on the basis of evoked potential data, the basic structures may be sensitive to verbal suggestions while later intentional processes, such as verbal rehearsal, are most certainly obliterated by anaesthetics.

Parallels exist in sleep research. A behavioural response to a verbal message administered to sleeping subjects was successfully carried out over adjacent and temporally remote sleep periods up to the 6-week period of the experiments. A suggestion followed by a cue word was spoken to highly suggestible subjects who were confirmed to be in stage 1 REM (rapid eye movement) sleep. The cue word elicited the suggested behaviour as confirmed by film records of subjects' sleep behaviour[20–22]. The sleep state was undisturbed during the learning and testing trials and was always stage 1 REM sleep. Subjects were amnesic for the suggestions, although sleep periods, tested days and even weeks later, confirmed that the verbal cue was still effective in eliciting the suggested behaviour. Memory enquiries included the use of hypnosis. In none of the subjects was hypnosis, or any other enquiry, able to reproduce the original suggestions which were nevertheless still behaviourally active. This indicates, by the late selection version of selective attention, that the knowledge base is at least partially located neurologically and temporally before conscious awareness *of* the event. Conscious awareness arises after knowledge has already intervened. Thus, the knowledge base can be activated *early* rather than *late* in the processing sequence. By this analysis, the late selection theory links with the sleep suggestion studies: effects of verbal suggestions were acted upon behaviourally (neurologically) by early, rather than by late, perceptual processes. Completely new information is not learned in these studies, rather existing knowledge is activated. Memory in terms of conscious recollection may indeed be amnesic when neurological processes act autonomously in early rather than late structures in the nervous system. Natural circadian sleep and general anaesthesia are not, however, the same. Rather, a behavioural response was demonstrated to verbal suggestions in the presence of a dense amnesia during the time when the effects of the suggestions were still active within the nervous system. This functional result is equivalent to what has been claimed for perception during general anaesthesia: post-anaesthetic effects in the presence of amnesia.

Therapeutic benefits[24,25] from positive suggestions addressed personally to anaesthetized surgical patients with direct physiological suggestions, but without a control group, were associated with doses of post-operative analgesics which were very small. Post-operative responses to minor surgical procedures were reportedly more successfully improved by intra-operative suggestion than were the outcomes to major surgery.

One study directed to the improvement of post-operative condition achieved earlier times to urination and the reduction in the need for a post-operative urinary catheter; eight of 12 controls required post-operative urinary catheterization; not one of the 12 suggestion patients did[13].

Studies by the author's group[4] utilized a personalized request that the patient indicate that they had heard the message by engaging in cued behaviour during the post-operative interview. Suggestion patients did so significantly more than controls by a 6:1 ratio. However, no patient verbally recalled the instruction given during anaesthesia, even during hypnosis. Personalized instructions were effective in demonstrating a cued response to verbal information presented during anaesthesia, for which the patient was amnesic.

An unpublished study was designed to test differences in auditory acquisition as a function of the duration of anaesthesia and the anaesthetic agents administered. A standardized, appropriate message was presented to patients during different phases of clinical anaesthesia and was followed by post-operative interviews which assessed verbal and non-verbal memories of the experimental message.

Forty-eight patients, ASA grades I–II, aged 19–63 years, scheduled for elective surgery were chosen (ASA = American Society of Anesthesiologists). Each consented to be a participant and institutional approval from the Human Subjects Review Committee was obtained. Patients were told that surgical personnel often assume that the patient does not record their conversations. The patient was told to listen for a special message during anaesthesia. To increase the meaningfulness of the neutral study message, patients were also told that a personal message for their good recovery would precede the study message. The interviewer made a tape recording for each patient which included the patient's preferred name, personalized statements of well-being regarding the specific operation, suggestions for recovery, and a statement on the importance of engaging in specific behaviour during a post-operative interview. The behaviour was randomly assigned among patients from four choices: touching the right or left ear, lifting the left or the right index finger.

Patients who required general anaesthesia for gastrointestinal, gynaecological, orthopaedic, or plastic surgery were studied. No attempt was made to control the anaesthetic technique. All patients received nitrous oxide 40–67% and isoflurane 0.25–1.5% ($n = 29$), halothane 0.5–2% ($n = 11$), or enflurane 1–3% ($n = 8$). Anaesthetic intravenous agents included sodium thiopentone, diazepam, fentanyl, and morphine sulphate. The anaesthetist confirmed that the patients were adequately anaesthetized and clinically stable. Heart rate and blood pressure did not change with the presentation of the message. All anaesthetic agents and their doses related to the time of message delivery were recorded. Presentation of the experimental message was through a tape recorder through stereo earphones fitted by a separate experimenter. This was monitored to ensure adequate presentation over a separate set of earphones. Post-operative interviews were conducted 1–20 days after anaesthesia. The two interviewers recorded all instances of the four non-verbal target behaviours throughout the 30-minute interview, at the end of which the entire taped message was played to the patient, breaking the blind condition for the experimenters. The presence or absence in the interview of the specific behaviour mentioned in the experimental message was taken as evidence for (or against) learning during general anaesthesia.

Pre- and intra-operative variables were recorded from patients. Doses of induction agents and anaesthetics, the time that the message was played to the patient after induction and before emergence, anaesthetics present at that time, pre- and intra-operative haemodynamics, and post-operative interview responses, including non-verbal responses, were recorded. A mathematical model (logistic regression) was developed from these data to determine which variables correlated with the presence of the suggested behaviour in the post-operative interview.

The results are given below.

Message presentation

The time of message presentation varied from 15 to 293 minutes after induction (10–219 minutes before emergence). The mean interval before the message was given was 93 minutes after intubation (s.d. 64.3 min) and 59 minutes before emergency (s.d. 58.2 min). The interview revealed that no patient verbally recalled the experimental message or any intra-operative event. Interview observation of patients' non-verbal behaviour revealed responses to the intra-operative message in 33 cases and a lack of a specific response in 15 cases.

The statistical model showed that two variables were associated with the post-operative non-verbal behaviour: presentation of the message for that response ($P < 0.02$), and a non-significant trend for intra-operative intravenous diazepam to suppress the response ($P = 0.13$). A noteworthy finding was a *lack of correlation* of time of presentation, levels of inhalational agents, or haemodynamic variables. The data suggest that *moment of presentation* does not modulate stimulus acquisition during anaesthesia. The results suggest a persistence of the acquisition of auditory information throughout adequate surgical anaesthesia. Patients' *verbal retrieval* abilities are therefore unreliable indicators of *sensory responses* to intra-operative auditory events. These results confirm neurophysiological findings of preservation of evoked auditory potentials throughout surgical anaesthesia. Statements during general anaesthesia which direct patient behaviour may, therefore, be effective despite post-operative verbal amnesia.

What is consciousness?

Consciousness, the word

From Latin, *conscio*, consciousness in its original form meant to know (*scio*) together with (*con*) another person: *con + scio = conscio*. This definition, the first definition of consciousness in the *Oxford English Dictionary*, is archaic and obsolete, though pertinent. Originally, a person was conscious only to the extent that he shared knowledge with another, especially in a private secretive way. In the Middle Ages, use of the word changed and split into two different meanings[26]. One branch retained the shared knowledge aspect of the term and became conscience: knowledge shared now with oneself, but not with others, as in a 'guilty conscience'.

Generic consciousness

The other branch of conscious became the generic form that medicine uses today, conscious as responsive to the environment[26]. This use misses several distinctions that are important to the issues of determining unconsciousness during general anaesthesia. It does not distinguish between registering information and being able to report what has been registered. It misses any electrophysiological distinctions relevant to the questions involving awareness, consciousness, and memory. It means simply that an outside observer sees movement more or less appropriate to instructions delivered to the patient to move (Open your eyes, Mr Smith, Can you hear me?, Take a deep breath).

The use of conscious by anaesthetists is similar to their use of the words aware and awake. The patient coming to after anaesthesia could be referred to by any of these words, but essentially their use indicates the patient can do something or move appropriately. Or the term could be applied to responding to a verbal request to the patient to open the eyes or squeeze a hand. Then, if there was an appropriate movement, the patient would be declared awake, aware, or conscious. If the apparently somnolent patient did not respond, a pain stimulus might be applied to the fingers or toes to arouse the patient. Here, a withdrawal or a verbal reaction to the stimulus would imply responsiveness and the terms again might be applied. For anaesthesia, conscious means observably responsive. This use of the word, it is claimed, results in confusion.

Consciousness, as shared knowledge

Returning to the original use of conscious, classic reports of 'awareness during anaesthesia' require the shared knowledge aspect of the word 'conscious' for qualification as awareness during anaesthesia: sharing with oneself the knowledge that one is aware, that is reflective consciousness. 'I am aware of X' (that surgery is occurring now) is sharing with oneself, alone, the ongoing sensations arriving at the brain. This ability to know that X is occurring, to be aware of X, is essentially to communicate with oneself that 'X is occurring'. Yet, as many data have shown, though lacking consciousness *of* X, X may still occur and affect the central nervous system with post-operative consequences. If particularly pertinent statements are made, these may activate reflective consciousness, as in the case reports of patients who apparently suddenly became aware when something important occurred.

Let us set the terms straight as they could be used in anaesthesia: consciousness is an aspect of mental activity which requires that there be reflective knowledge – knowledge about X sensation, thought, or feeling. This quality of mental life is inferred by the patient's report or behaviour. The patient states that there was an event X of which he was conscious. Consciousness is known in the first person.

Awareness is the observation of responsiveness. A patient may move on incision, respond to a command, receive a communication in a drowsy state which acts later like a posthypnotic suggestion, withdraw from a pain stimulus, or simply be assessed as responsive to the environment; these observations of the patient lead us to consider that the patient is aware, but the patient may lack the reflective capacity to appreciate that he is experiencing the event and nearly always lacks the ability to report later about these events, that is to state verbally that he was conscious. Awareness is thus a judgement made by an outside observer, based on the patient's behaviour, while consciousness is a quality of mental life known only by the patient and then reported to others. Awareness, by this use, must also extend to other life forms which are also responsive to the environment, but consciousness can only be known by interacting with an individual or an individual interacting with himself, that is aware of his sensory input. In terms of the 'last to go' function of audition, a guess on how this occurs would involve reticular activating system activation to pertinent auditory stimulation, and would be positively related to the degree of importance of the signal that was activated in the knowledge base of long-term memory. Thus, adequate anaesthesia would be adequate until particularly important information was present, during which time there would be attempts to bring reticular activating system activity to bear on the information, which could produce reflective consciousness ('awareness'), or could simply produce memories inaccessible to consciousness.

By a model of automatic analysis of semantic information[27, 28], the central nervous system would preferentially respond to pertinent information – relevant to survival and well-being – rather than information irrelevant to those concerns. Learning, non-verbal memory, affective and vegetative systems, and stress physiology are potential targets of both supportive information and, regrettably, derogatory or pessimistic information. Similarly, it is conceivable that alerting information could activate centres which mediate consciousness, and thus induce an awareness during anaesthesia where none would have been present. This would apply only to those cases where delivery of anaesthesia was well documented, yet the patient still reported accurate recall.

The nature of processing information, especially language, during anaesthesia depends on automatically activating the knowledge base in long-term memory. It is clear now from cognitive psychology that semantic analysis can occur well in advance of consciousness of that message[27]. Thus, in addition to understanding that pertinent information activates early knowledge structures, anaesthetists should recognize that these activations are not benign but can in both positive and negative instances have intellectually interesting and clinically important consequences.

References

1. WEINBERGER, N. M., GOLD, P. E. and STERNBERG, D. B. (1984) Epinephrine enables Pavlovian fear conditioning under anesthesia. *Science*, **223**, 605–607
2. LEVINSON, B. W. (1969) An examination of states of awareness during general anaesthesia. *Doctoral Thesis*, University of the Witwatersrand, South Africa
3. EICH, E., REEVES, J. L. and KATZ, R. L. (1985) Anesthesia, amnesia and the memory/awareness distinction. *Anesthesia and Analgesia*, **64**, 1143–1148
4. BENNETT, H. L., DAVIS, H. S. and GIANNINI, J. A. (1985) Non-verbal response to intraoperative conversation. *British Journal of Anaesthesia*, **57**, 174–179
5. GOLDMANN, L. (1986) Awareness under general anaesthesia. *PhD Thesis*, Cambridge University, Cambridge, England
6. KUMAR, S. M., PANDIT, S. K. and JACKSON, P. F. (1978) Recall following ketamine anesthesia for open-heart surgery: report of a case. *Anesthesia and Analgesia*, **57**, 267–269

7. HILGENBERG, J. C. (1981) Intraoperative awareness during high-dose fentanyl–oxygen anesthesia. *Anesthesiology,* **54**, 341–343

8. SAUCIER, N., WALTS, L. F. and MORELAND, J. R. (1983) Patient awareness during nitrous oxide, oxygen, and halothane anesthesia. *Anesthesia and Analgesia,* **62**, 239–240

9. RATH, B. (1982) The use of suggestions during general anaesthesia. *Doctoral Dissertation,* University of Louisville, Kentucky, USA

10. TRUSTMAN, R., DUBOVSKY, S. and TITLEY, R. (1977) Auditory perception during general anaesthesia – myth or fact? *International Journal of Clinical and Experimental Hypnosis,* **25**, 88–105

11. BITNER, R. L. (1983) Awareness during anesthesia. In *Complications in Anesthesiology,* edited by F. K. Orkin and L. H. Cooperman. Philadelphia: J. B. Lippincott Co.

12. BLACHER, R. S. (1984) Awareness during surgery (Editorial). *Anesthesiology,* **61**, 1–2

13. MAINORD, W. A., RATH, B. and BARNETT, F. (1983) Anesthesia and suggestion. Paper presented at American Psychological Annual Convention, 1983, Los Angeles, California

14. MILLAR, K. and WATKINSON, N. (1983) Recognition of words presented during general anaesthesia. *Ergonomics,* **26**, 585–594

15. BONKE, B., SCHMITZ, P. I. M., VERHAGE, F. and ZWAVELING, A. (1984) A clinical study of so-called unconscious perception during general anesthesia. *British Journal of Anaesthesia,* **58**, 957–964

16. LOFTUS, E. F., SCHOOLER, J. W., LOFTUS, G. R. and GLAUBER, D. T. (1985) Memory for events occurring under anesthesia. *Acta Psychologica,* **59**, 123–128

17. STOLZY, S., COUTURE, L. J. and EDMONDS, H. L. JR (1986) Evidence of partial recall during general anesthesia. *Anesthesia and Analgesia,* **65**, S154

18. ADAM, N. (1979) Disruption of memory functions associated with general anesthetics. In *Functional Disorders of Memory,* edited by J. F. Kihlstrom and F. J. Evans. Hillsdale, New Jersey: Lawrence Erlbaum Association

19. YEAKEL, A. E. (1974) Recall of events while under general anesthesia. *Pennsylvania Medicine,* **77**, 47–49

20. EVANS, F. J., GUSTAFSON, L. A., O'CONNELL, D. N., ORNE, M. T. and SHOR, R. E. (1966) Response during sleep with intervening waking amnesia. *Science,* **152**, 666–667

21. EVANS, F. J., GUSTAFSON, L. A., O'CONNELL, D. N., ORNE, M. T. and SHOR, R. E. (1969) Sleep-induced behavioral response. Relationship to susceptibility to hypnosis and laboratory sleep patterns. *Journal of Nervous and Mental Disease,* **148**, 467–476

22. EVANS, F. (1979) Hypnosis and sleep: Techniques for exploring cognitive activity during sleep. In *Hypnosis: Developments in Research and New Perspectives,* 2nd edn, edited by E. Fromm and R. E. Shor, pp. 139–183. New York: Aldine Publ. Co.

23. PERRY, C. W., EVANS, F. J., O'CONNEL, D. N., ORNE, E. and ORNE, M. T. (1978) Behavioral response to verbal stimuli administered and tested during REM sleep: a further investigation. *Waking and Sleeping,* **2**, 35–42

24. HUTCHINGS, D. D. (1961) The value of suggestion given under anesthesia: a report and evaluation of 200 consecutive cases. *American Journal of Clinical Hypnosis,* **4**, 26–29

25. WOLFE, L. S. and MILLET, J. B. (1960) Control of post-operative pain by suggestion under general anesthesia. *American Journal of Clinical Hypnosis,* **3**, 109–112

26. LEWIS, C. S. (1967) *Studies in Words.* Cambridge: The University Press

27. DIXON, N. (1981) *Preconscious Processing.* New York: John Wiley and Sons

28. BENNETT, H. L. (1980) Selective Attention: The expression of suggested actions in an unattended message. *Doctoral Dissertation,* University of California, Davis

Chapter 16

Further evidence for cognitive processing under general anaesthesia

L. Goldmann

Bennett (*see* Chapter 15) presented studies which demonstrated that patients may perform, post-operatively, non-verbal acts in response to intra-operative suggestions without recall, either of the suggestion or phenomenal awareness of their responses to it. The research presented in this chapter supports Bennett's findings. In addition, a wider range of post-operative responses is examined. A key variable in these responses is their degree of intentionality. The evidence is drawn from experimental studies of orienting responses, post-operative non-verbal responses, recognition, and recall. All of the patients involved in the studies were elective surgical patients. The following points need to be discussed: evidence for cognitive processing depends upon how it is defined and how it is measured; the historical reliance upon recall as a measure of memory has led to the erroneous belief that patients do not recollect intra-operative events; and evidence for recollection of intra-operative events decreases as the intentionality of retrieval strategies increases.

Previous writings concerning memory for events which occurred while a patient was thought to have been adequately anaesthetized have relied predominantly upon the term 'awareness' and have used it synonomously with recall. This is unfortunate, because being aware of something is not the same as being able to bring it intentionally to mind. The term 'awareness' has been used to describe events as disparate as verbatim recall of intra-operative conversation accompanied by paralysis and pain, as well as post-operative non-verbal responses to intra-operative suggestions (*see* Chapter 15).

The association of the term 'awareness' with recall has led to the use of the term 'cognitive processing' in this circumstance. Evidence for cognitive processing under anaesthesia includes any psychologically mediated response which occurs during or after the operation, and which can be said to have been elicited by an intra-operative event.

The case against recall

Recall is but one measure of recollection. Few researchers have been able to record adequately positive instances of recall with all the necessary experimental safeguards (for example, Levinson was not blind to the intra-operative event). Consequently, the dominant belief in anaesthetic practice has been that the encoding of information under adequate general anaesthesia and its subsequent retrieval is a rare event. An alternative view is that recall is simply a poor measure to assess cognitive processing under anaesthesia.

Less intentional measures of recollection (recognition or spelling) or those that tap skill or procedural memories (learning a puzzle or riding a bicycle) are less vulnerable to state-dependent variables, such as drugs, context, and specific memory impairments, such as Korsakoff's syndrome. Furthermore, recall usually involves a social interaction. How a patient is interviewed, the questions asked, by whom, and with what perceived consequences, can dramatically influence how, whether, and with what degree of accuracy an event is recalled. Even if the interview situation were to be ideal, the meaning for the patient of being able to recall an intra-operative event may influence how and whether it is reported.

Anaesthesia is not sleep, and intra-operative events are not dreams, but it may be useful to mention those factors that influence the recall of dreams. These are the salience and content of the dream, medication administered prior to sleep, the manner in which the dreamer is awakened, the context in which the dream is dreamt, the personality characteristics of the dreamer, and the demand characteristics of the post-dream interview: all factors which could reasonably influence the recall of intra-operative events. A dreamer may wish to recall a dream, but a patient may have good reasons for wanting to forget an intra-operative event.

A dreamer may not be able to recall his dream, but he may be left with the impression that he dreamt. Here the failure to recall does not imply that the event 'dreaming' did not occur. External stimuli may be incorporated in dreams. A barking dog may become a roaring lion. The dreamer may also be left with emotions or thoughts arising from the dream which he may or may not be able to explain or attribute to the dream. In a similar manner, surgical patients may have feelings, thoughts, or associations which he may or may not attribute to intra-operative events.

For example, after induction, while a patient was still in the anaesthetic room, an anaesthetist explained to a medical student about the muscle contractions which followed the use of methohexitone. The anaesthetist observed that this was very much like what he had seen when bodies were placed upon the funeral pyres in India. The following morning, the patient reported that he had had a hot and restless night's sleep. He felt agitated but did not recall any event between induction and waking in the recovery room. There is a plausible connection between these two events. It cannot be proven. This instance does, however, suggest the subtlety and type of evidence that may predominate when recollection of intra-operative events is investigated. Here the salience of the event and the affective, non-verbal nature of the response are important factors. Less dramatic, but possibly more persuasive, data are found cited below.

Some support for information processing under general anaesthesia can be found from responses to intra-operative stimuli which resulted in orienting responses[1] (EEGs[1],), non-verbal responses in the form of affect[2], specific behavioural responses[3], classic conditioning (in animals) demonstrated by response suppression[4], recognition of words using a signal detection task[5], recall of operative events through dream-like processes[6], and verbatim recall[1,7].

The following studies were all conducted by the author and reproduce some of the above findings. The studies proceed from the least to the most intentional forms of remembering: orienting, non-verbal responses, recognition, and recall. All patients, with the exception of those participating in the orienting study, were given an extensive pre-operative interview. In addition to informing and relaxing the patient, one function of the interview was to engage the patient's interest by suggesting the possible beneficial aspects of the studies. All of the taped messages began with the patient's name, included a positive suggestion of the patient's choice (giving up smoking), a suggestion designed to be experimentally tested, and a suggestion for a quick and easy recovery. The effectiveness of the patient's chosen suggestion was not assessed.

Orienting

The orienting response or 'investigatory reflex' can be elicited by stimuli that are novel, surprising, complex, or emotional. The salience of the stimulus can be influenced by expectation and motivation. In order for a stimulus to be considered salient, it must be compared to elements in short or long-term memory as well as to pre-existing cognitive sets and hypotheses. Consequently, a degree of encoding, matching and retrieval of information must occur.

Two studies were conducted to assess orienting responses in premedicated spontaneously breathing patients receiving nitrous oxide and halothane[8]. In the first series, the majority of a sample of patients from whom a galvanic skin response could be obtained, showed an orienting response when a name thought to be highly salient was mentioned: the leader of the National Union of Mineworkers during the time of the mineworker's strike. Other stimuli which were thought to be salient, such as the patient's name or remarks regarding the surgery, did not necessarily elicit an orienting response. This underlines the notion that remarks thought to be salient may or may not be important for the patient. In a second series, galvanic skin responses were elicited significantly more often ($P < 0.01$) to recorded sounds and statements than to recorded silence.

Post-operative non-verbal behaviour

A similar procedure as described by Bennett in Chapter 15 was used to assess memory for intra-operative suggestions in cardiac patients undergoing cardiopulmonary bypass and receiving a narcotic anaesthetic[9]. The suggestion was given to patients after the end of bypass and were rewarmed to 37 °C. A randomly selected group of patients was requested to touch their chin during a post-operative interview. Those patients who had been asked to touch their chin did so significantly more often ($P < 0.01$) than the control group.

Recognition

Significantly higher recognition scores ($P < 0.01$) for information presented under anaesthesia were found in a group of spontaneously breathing patients who received nitrous oxide, oxygen and halothane versus controls who received the same pre-operative preparation but with a different taped message. All patients were administered a pre-operative test which included obscure questions of the nature 'What is the blood pressure of an octopus?'. Of those patients whose performance improved from pre-test to post-test, few guessed that they had been given the answers during their operation. One patient explained his improved performance by saying: 'There is just more in my head than there was before'.

Recall

The following three studies give additional support to the notion that evidence for recall, even when efforts are made to maximize its occurrence, is difficult to find and may be uncovered at risk of psychological distress to the patient.

Returning to the study of cardiac patients mentioned above, seven of the 30 patients (23%) reported recall. Three of these reports (10%) included either verbatim recall of conversations which were later corroborated or information which the patient could not have known beforehand. Less pre-operative medication (< 0.01) and higher post-operative anxiety ($P < 0.05$) were the best predictors of those patients reporting recall. The interviews were conducted 7–10 days post-operatively. All patients who reported recall became anxious during their interviews, some markedly so.

In a double-blind trial which involved premedicated spontaneously breathing patients receiving nitrous oxide, oxygen and halothane, little evidence for recall was found when intra-operative stimuli of low and moderate salience were played to the patients. Information thought to be salient to the patient was gleaned during the pre-operative interview. Of 25 patients, three reported images that could be associated with the taped message.

(a) *Taped message:* You have a lovely garden.
    Interviewer (I)   Does anything else come to mind?
    Patient (P)   Tomatoes and lettuce.
    (I)   Anything about tomatoes and lettuce?
    (P)   We are trying to grow them in our garden.
(b) You left nursing to have a lovely little girl.
    (I) Does anything come to mind that was said to you or about you in theatre?
    (P) No. I am just thinking about my family.

These messages were designed not to stress the patient. The patient's hearing was not completely occluded during operation so intra-operative events, which were of greater salience, may have overshadowed the pre-recorded messages.

In a third study, the experimenter was not blind to the intra-operative stimulus. All patients were women and all good hypnotic subjects. The same suggestion was used throughout: 'When you awaken from your anaesthetic, you will believe for a moment that you have green hair.' The statements of three patients are suggestive of the taped message. The excerpt from the first interview occurred under hypnosis.

(a) (I) Anything at all. Anything come to mind?
    (P) Well, I dreamt of green strands.
(b) (I) Does anything come to mind when you think about your operation?
    (P) No.
    (I) What about now? Anything at all?
    (P) I keep thinking about green things.
(c) (I) How are you this morning?
    (P) Pretty good.
    (I) Everything went well?
    (P) Great, I'm leaving this morning. I can't wait to wash my hair.

Clearly, even the use of an informed interviewer, good hypnotic subjects, and hypnosis (which may improve rapport, and help reinstate context) does not supply incontrovertible evidence for recall. Recall is decidedly not a good measure of whether information has been processed under general anaesthesia. This is supported by research with subclinical doses of inhalational anaesthetics which suggests that encoding and retrieval of verbal information is particularly disrupted[10].

Recall may thus be a poor measure of memory for intra-operative events, but persuasive evidence can be found by examining emotional responses, non-verbal behaviour, associations, and desires. These behavioural patterns are often subtle, unnoticed by staff, open to interpretation, and difficult to investigate. These difficulties should not prevent researchers from finding additional evidence that patients hear and are influenced by what they hear under general anaesthesia. We might, therefore, begin to think of suggestions which could improve the patient's welfare.

References

1. LEVINSON, B. W. (1965) States of awareness during general anaesthesia. Preliminary communication. *British Journal of Anaesthesia*, **37**, 544–546
2. BLACHER, R. S. (1975) On awakening paralyzed during surgery. A syndrome of traumatic neurosis. *Journal of the American Medical Association*, **234**, 67–68
3. BENNETT, H. L., DAVIS, H. S. and GIANNINI, J. A. (1985) Non-verbal response to intraoperative conversation. *British Journal of Anaesthesia*, **57**, 174–179
4. WEINBERGER, N. M., GOLD, P. E. and STERNBERG, D. B. (1984) Epinephrine enables Pavlovian fear conditioning under anesthesia. *Science*, **223**, 605–606
5. MILLAR, K. and WATKINSON, N. (1983) Recognition of words presented during general anaesthesia. *Ergonomics*, **26**, 585–594
6. FEDERN, P. (1953) A dream under general anaesthesia. In *Ego Psychology and the Psychoses*, edited by P. Federn, pp. 100–104. London: Imago Pub. Co.
7. CHEEK, D. B. (1959) Unconscious perception of meaningful sounds during surgical anesthesia as revealed under hypnosis. *American Journal of Clinical Hypnosis*, **1**, 101–113
8. GOLDMANN, L. and LEVEY, A. B. (1986) Orientating under anaesthesia. *Anaesthesia*, **41**, 1056–1057
9. GOLDMANN, L., SHAH, M. and HEBDEN, M. (1987) Memory and cardiac anaesthesia. *Anaesthesia*, **42** (in press)
10. ADAM, N. (1979) Disruption of memory functions associated with general anaesthetics. In *Functional Disorders of Memory*, edited by J. F. Kilstrom and F. J. Evans, pp. 219–238. Hillsdale, NJ: Lawrence Ellbaum Association

Chapter 17

Testing for memory of events during anaesthesia

P. J. Standen

When a general anaesthetic is administered, the anaesthetist aims to keep the patient unresponsive to painful stimulation and amnesic for the period of anaesthesia. Most attempts to prevent these two experiences depend upon monitoring the patient for changes associated with the possibility of later reports of awareness.

However, as far as amnesia is concerned, it may result from a failure to register incoming information or through a failure to make the registered information available to consciousness at a later time. Even under adequate anaesthesia, the auditory system still registers incoming information[1] and experiments on laboratory subjects demonstrate that conscious attention at presentation is not necessary for material to influence behaviour at a later date[2]. Monitoring systems designed to detect events, which will correlate with or predict subsequent reports of awareness, may blind us to the fact that there is no truly obtunded state. It may be possible to correlate these with a sensation of pain but not with the registering of incoming information.

However, if auditory information is registered when the patient is less than fully conscious, it may have a reduced likelihood of re-entering awareness than if the individual was fully attentive at the time of registration. Full attention may allow the integration of the event with existing memories thus generating associations which facilitate retrieval[3].

Re-entering awareness can take place in a variety of different ways. A witness to a robbery may be able to provide a detailed, unprompted account in response to the question 'What did you see?'. On the other hand, he or she may be unable to describe the getaway car unless prompted by questions of the type 'Was it a saloon/foreign car?'. Alternatively, the witness may only be able to recognize the vehicle if given a choice of pictures of possible cars. If all three approaches produce blanks, it is possible that at a later date the image of the getaway car may 'pop-up' into consciousness when the witness has not even been considering the event. The better formed the memory is, in the sense of its integration with other stored material, the more likely is unprompted recall.

Memory for events during anaesthesia is unlikely to be demonstrated by unprompted recall and many studies have failed using direct questioning. It therefore follows that other techniques must be utilized, especially if it is believed that the memory was stored during a state of reduced consciousness.

Jones and Konieczko[4] emphasize that the information registered during anaesthesia is held in long-term memory, is wholly unconscious and probably cannot be retrieved into working memory. Bennett, Davis and Giannini[5] proposed that hypnosis might provide a possible interface to access otherwise dissociated (i.e. difficult to retrieve) memory structures of events during general anaesthesia. Hypnosis has been employed to improve recall of crimes or events of legal significance. However, in this field, warnings have been issued[6,7] that any pressure to enhance recall beyond the initial attempt may increase the number of errors as well as correct recall. Hypnosis exaggerates this process, particularly so for those with hypnotic susceptibility. Material elicited under hypnosis is also difficult to quantify objectively. Interestingly, Bennett, Davis and Giannini[5] found no recall under hypnosis of an instruction given during general anaesthesia, although this instruction appeared to later influence behaviour in their experimental group.

If we are worried about auditory material registering during anaesthesia and influencing a patient's later behaviour, for example, detrimental remarks which delay recovery[8,9], it follows that we must test for this by examining subsequent changes in a patient, related to the material to which they are exposed while anaesthetized. For example, in one study during anaesthesia, the patient received a suggestion to touch the ear during a subsequent interview[5]. Hutchings[8] suggested that, if the patient's later behaviour could be influenced by intra-operative suggestion, this could be exploited to improve their recovery.

There are other techniques which may be simpler to quantify than these. Goldmann (Chapter 16) reports a study where, during anaesthesia, patients were given answers to questions which, prior to surgery, they had not known. This procedure increased their performance on retest post-operatively over that of a group that had not received this information.

Another approach is to utilize techniques usually associated with the testing of amnesic patients. These subjects show some similarity to those considered here because neither can they verbally retrieve test material, nor do they have any memory of being exposed to the material in the first place. Spontaneous recall or direct questioning may give an impression of a totally oblivious patient during anaesthesia. Yet these particular techniques have always demonstrated poor memory in amnesiacs when other techniques have elicited some memory trace. Warrington and Weiskrantz[10], testing amnesic patients, found that, although their recognition of recently exposed words was notoriously poor, their recall approached the level shown by normals if they were cued by the first three letters of the learned word.

Meudell and Mayes[11] used the same technique with normals and also recorded subjects' ratings of how confident they were of the correctness of their answers. They found that confidence ratings were negatively related to recall. Subjects were tested at 15 minutes and 6 weeks after exposure to test material and, if only the correct responses were considered, they were more confident about them at 15 minutes than at 6 weeks. In other words, at 6 weeks they did not think that they knew, but they did.

Considering that this may be similar to the situation in which post-anaesthetic patients find themselves, the author's group[12] used a type of cued recall to test for the registration of auditory material to which patients were exposed during anaesthesia. Children who had routine surgery received, over headphones, a tape-recorded message including six words to which they were instructed to attend. Post-operatively they were tested with cues that were shared by more than one word, and the words that were less common (as determined by a pilot study) were the ones played during anaesthesia.

It was expected, as in the study by Stolzy, Couture and Edmonds[13], that by the use of uncommon words during anaesthesia, subjects cued post-operatively, who had heard the words, were more likely to produce these uncommon words than subjects who had not heard the words. The tape was played to two groups of subjects who differed only in the level of anaesthesia (in terms of the percentage of halothane breathed). The cued recall test was given to an additional group who had not heard the tape. The 'light' group produced more items than did the other two groups, but this difference was only significant ($P < 0.05$) when it was compared with the other group who had heard the tape. All groups were similar in their responsiveness at the time of testing. If this type of testing is to make a valuable contribution to the evaluation of unconsciousness, then there are two aspects of the design of this study on which it is important to focus attention. The first is the nature of the message played over headphones. Most laboratory experiments on selective attention use neutral material, although in a dichotic listening task subjects will switch to the untracked channel if a stimulus of high relevance (like the subject's name) occurs.

With the exception of the study by Levinson[9], neutral material is also used in studies of anaesthetized patients and this may account for the negative results that are found. One attempt to increase the pertinence of the material without involving ethical considerations is to preface the message with the patient's name. This method was used in the author's study. Millar and Watkinson[14] suggest using organized verbal material. A laboratory experiment[15] found that words presented in context were more likely to be detected.

A second aspect for consideration is the interval between recovery from anaesthesia and the time of the test. Studies with positive findings are those where testing took place later, either within 48 hours[13] or within 24 hours[14]. When no effect was found[16], testing occurred as soon after surgery as possible. In the present study, patients were tested within 24 hours, primarily because they were discharged soon after. Today's short-stay admissions make late testing difficult but crucial. Evidence from studies of serial reaction-time[17] suggests that psychological functioning may take up to 48 hours to return to pre-anaesthetic levels. Adam[18] presents evidence that retrieval from memory of material learned under the effect of anaesthetic agents, depending on type of material, shows a better performance at one week after learning than at 2 hours.

Testing for some memory of events during anaesthesia gives an account of the patient's level of consciousness when it is too late. If attention is paid to the design of those techniques they could be combined with the methods of monitoring described in earlier chapters to increase knowledge of when a patient is at risk of registering events in theatre.

It would be unwise to decide that the occurrence of this registration always indicated an inadequate level of anaesthesia. The obvious benefits of new anaesthesia techniques with muscle relaxants and local blocks are not to be abandoned for fear of the patient hearing something. Hearing, in itself, is not such a harmful experience. Blacher[19] commented that the patient who was very much awake was better off. Indeed, some surgery is carried out with merely a local anaesthetic when the patient remains capable of hearing everything in theatre. Perhaps it should be acknowledged that some hearing may always occur and attention turned towards preventing this from being an unpleasant experience for the patient.

References

1. WINTERS, W. D. (1976) Effects of drugs on the electrical activity of the brain: anesthetics. *Annual Review of Pharmacology and Toxicology,* **16**, 413–426
2. EICH, E. (1984) Memory for unattended events: remembering with and without awareness. *Memory and Cognition,* **12**, 105–111
3. UNDERWOOD, G. (1979) Memory systems and conscious processes. In *Aspects of Consciousness,* Vol. 1, edited by G. Underwood and R. Stevens, pp. 91–121. London: Academic Press
4. JONES, J. G. and KONIECZKO, K. (1986) Hearing and memory in anaesthetized patients. *British Medical Journal,* **292**, 1291–1293
5. BENNETT, H. L., DAVIS, H. S. and GIANNINI, J. A. (1985) Non-verbal response to intraoperative conversation. *British Journal of Anaesthesia,* **57**, 174–179
6. DYWAN, J. and BOWERS, K. (1983) The use of hypnosis to enhance recall. *Science,* **222**, 184–185
7. LAURENCE, J. R. and PERRY, C. (1983) Hypnotically created memory among highly hypnotizable subjects. *Science,* **222**, 523–524
8. HUTCHINGS, D. D. (1961) The value of suggestion given under anesthesia: report and evaluation of 200 consecutive cases. *American Journal of Clinical Hypnosis,* **4**, 26–29
9. LEVINSON, B. W. (1965) States of awareness during general anaesthesia. Preliminary communication. *British Journal of Anaesthesia,* **37**, 544–546
10. WARRINGTON, E. K. and WEISKRANTZ, L. (1974) The effect of prior learning on subsequent retention in amnesic patients. *Neuropsychologica,* **12**, 419–428
11. MEUDELL, P. R. and MAYES, A. R. (1984) Patterns of confidence loss in the cued recall of normal people with attenuated recognition memory: their relevance to a similar amnesic phenomenon. *Neuropsychologica,* **22**, 41–54
12. STANDEN, P. J., HAIN, W. R. and HOSKER, K. J. (1987) Retention of auditory information presented during anaesthesia. *Anaesthesia,* **42**, 604–608
13. STOLZY, S., COUTURE, L. J. and EDMONDS, H. L. (1986) Evidence of partial recall during general anesthesia. *Anesthesia and Analgesia,* **65**, S154
14. MILLAR, K. and WATKINSON, N. (1983) Recognition of words presented during general anaesthesia. *Ergonomics,* **26**, 585–594
15. TREISMAN, A. and GEFFEN, G. (1968) Selective attention: perception or response? *Quarterly Journal of Experimental Psychology,* **19**, 1–17
16. DUBOVSKY, S. L. and TRUSTMAN, R. (1976) Absence of recall after general anesthesia: implications for theory and practice. *Anesthesia and Analgesia,* **55**, 696–701
17. HERBERT, M., HEALY, T. E. J., BOURKE, J. B., FLETCHER, I. R. and ROSE, J. M. (1983) Profile of recovery after general anaesthesia. *British Medical Journal,* **286**, 1539–1542
18. ADAM, N. (1979) Disruption of memory functions associated with general anesthetics. In *Functional Disorders of Memory,* edited by J. F. Kihlstrom and F. J. Evans, pp. 219–338. Hillsdale, New Jersey: Lawrence Erlbaum Association
19. BLACHER, R. S. (1984) Awareness during surgery (Editorial). *Anesthesiology,* **61**, 1–2

Chapter 18

Awareness: a medicolegal problem

R. L. Hargrove

A patient, who signs a consent form and agrees to have an operation performed under general anaesthesia, expects to be unconscious and free from pain or unpleasant sensations during the surgical procedure. He or she does not anticipate hearing a surgeon and assistant conversing while they work. Yet, since the advent of muscle relaxant drugs and their introduction to anaesthetic practice in the 1940s, the possibility of a paralysed patient remaining awake has become a reality; fortunately a very uncommon experience but one that in recent years is seemingly on the increase. A number of cases have been reported from time to time, but for the last 15 years the Medical Defence Union (MDU) has received an average of four or five cases per year.

In 1985, a patient in Wigan sued her anaesthetist because she was awake during a caesarean section. The facts of the case were very much in her favour so that damages in excess of £13 000 were awarded to her and the whole affair attracted considerable publicity. As a result, a whole series of claims were made by patients that they, too, had been awake during various surgical procedures. Public realization of a potential hazard of a medical procedure frequently leads to an increase in claims against doctors and not all the claims are related to events in recent years. A number inevitably are made for events that occurred many years, perhaps even decades, previously. Claims of awareness during general anaesthesia have been made for events that occurred as long ago as 1979 after the Wigan case. The Statute of Limitations, in theory, bars a plaintiff from making a first claim for events that occurred more than 3 years previously, but in practice it is not difficult for this limitation to be overcome.

An anaesthetist would do well to reflect that a patient who claims to have been awake during an operation is very likely to be correct. Some such claims are undoubtedly spurious, while others may be based upon a hazy recollection of immediate post-anaesthetic dreams or other para-operative phenomena. Most claims, particularly those which detail severe pain or discomfort, the inability to breathe or awareness of the noise of their surroundings, carry the ring of truth. Frequently, a patient's subsequent complaints and recollection of events in the operating theatre can be verified in detail, by those who are present at the time.

An increase in number of genuine claims by patients of awareness during general anaesthesia very probably bears some relationship to the current anaesthetic practice of supplementing nitrous oxide and oxygen anaesthesia with intravenous narcotic drugs, rather than inhalational agents. Adequate doses of narcotic analgesics usually ensure that a patient is pain free, but they do not offer a certainty that a patient will be unaware, least of all when the ratio of oxygen to nitrous oxide is more than 30%.

It is too frequently assumed that awareness during general anaesthesia is restricted to obstetric anaesthetic practice. Such cases figure prominently in litigation, but they account for only 28% of all the cases of awareness reported to the Medical Defence Union. Anaesthesia for general surgical procedures accounted for 31% of cases, and a further 18% involved patients undergoing gynaecological procedures. There were 11% of cases associated with orthopaedic operations and the remaining 12% of cases were associated with dental, otolaryngological and ophthalmological operations. It is clear that most cases of reported awareness occurred in situations where there were no requirements for a minimal level of analgesia.

Reasons for awareness during general anaesthesia

The cases reported to the Medical Defence Union can be classified according to the probable reason for the awake state.

Faulty anaesthetic technique

The majority of cases (70%) fall into this category and most of these are where the anaesthetist has relied upon the nitrous oxide:oxygen:narcotic sequence to ensure unconsciousness. This may result in awareness in a proportion of cases. When a volatile agent has been used, it has either been in too small a concentration or has only been used intermittently during the anaesthetic. In caesarean section cases, it seems common practice to give a small dose of thiopentone (3.5 mg/kg) or methohexitone (1 mg/kg) followed by suxamethonium. The patient's lungs are ventilated with a 50% mixture of nitrous oxide and oxygen after tracheal intubation until the baby is delivered. Frequently, after delivery, if a narcotic is given, it is a very small dose and no allowance is made for the time it takes for an intravenous dose to act. There seems to be a reluctance, on the part of junior anaesthetists in particular, to use a volatile supplement such as 0.5% halothane in the period between induction of anaesthesia and delivery of the baby. The greatest risk of awareness occurs in this period. There is no good evidence to show that babies born to mothers having only nitrous oxide and oxygen are in a better condition than those where the mother has had a volatile agent given as part of the technique. Indeed, it is possible that if the mother is awake during the operation the result of the increased catecholamine output could easily result in delivery of a baby who is in a worse, rather than a better, state. When the caesarean section is being performed for severe fetal distress, some anaesthetists might feel that very light anaesthesia is justified but, again, there is no good evidence to show that such a technique is to the advantage of the baby or to the mother. If the anaesthetist really believes that very light anaesthesia is justified, then he must ensure that the patient is fully acquainted with the possibility of being aware. If he does not inform the patient of this possibility, and the patient subsequently sues, it makes it much more difficult to defend him on a charge of negligence. Another group of patients who are at risk from a faulty technique are those admitted as day cases. They are usually unpremedicated and given small doses of a short-acting induction agent, sometimes followed by a relaxant. Unless great care is taken in ventilating these patients' lungs with a gas mixture that ensures unconsciousness, awareness occurs in a number of cases. There is a tendency to intubate the trachea, paralyse and ventilate patients' lungs when the indication for such a technique does not exist. Patients having operations which require little or no relaxation seldom require paralysis, and controlled ventilation of the lungs may need volatile or other supplement to maintain reflex inactivity. Fewer orthopaedic cases would come to litigation if this fact were appreciated. Patients have also been awake due to the inattention of the anaesthetist or his absence from the operating theatre altogether. Such episodes are unforgivable and indefensible.

Finally, difficult tracheal intubation is a common cause of temporary awareness. If the dose of induction agent is small and difficulties arise, there is a tendency to give the patient more relaxant without an additional dose of induction agent. This particularly applies to caesarean sections. Such a technique inevitably results in the patient being aware of the attempted intubation and there have been several graphic accounts of what it feels like to have a laryngoscopy and attempted intubation while awake and paralysed.

Failure to check apparatus

Twenty per cent of cases of awareness are the direct result of the anaesthetist failing to check his anaesthetic apparatus. Difficulties arise when the connection between the anaesthetic machine and the ventilator is loose or completely disconnected. The patient can then under certain circumstances be ventilated with room air alone and is wide awake and in pain. It is surprising that the anaesthetist involved does not notice the increase in blood pressure and pulse rate, the sweating, or lacrimation.

In some cases the emergency oxygen control was left on and the gases were diluted to the extent that the patient could not possibly be unconscious. Checking of the apparatus would have overcome these difficulties.

Cases of awareness have arisen as a result of the vaporizer not being correctly locked on the back bar of the anaesthetic machine. In other cases, flexible connections to the vaporizer have been detached through back pressure or failure to check the security of the tapered fittings. Disconnections, partial or complete, account for other cases in this section and the message must be that a check of the anaesthetic apparatus before every case is essential.

Genuine apparatus failure

When part of the anaesthetic apparatus fails, and this could not have been detected by a diligent anaesthetist using the normal methods of testing prior to the start of the anaesthetic, then this can be considered a genuine apparatus failure. Vaporizers which deliver concentrations of vapour well below that indicated by the dial setting are included under this heading. Ventilators have been known to malfunction and to allow the patient to be ventilated with low concentrations of nitrous oxide. Here again, an anaesthetist could not be expected to detect the fault in the apparatus although he should perhaps be able to recognize the signs of light anaesthesia. The manufacturers of faulty apparatus would usually be expected to contribute to any damages awarded in such a case.

Spurious claim

Publicity surrounding cases of awareness undoubtedly generates an attitude in some members of the general public that money can be obtained by merely stating that awareness has taken place. This, in the eyes of the law, is insufficient to constitute a case of negligence against the anaesthetist. When these patients are asked for more details of the awareness, it soon becomes evident that such an event did not take place and the claim is entirely spurious. These cases can be contested and are often withdrawn before they reach the courts. The number of cases that fall into this category is 2.5%.

Justified risks

When a patient is desperately ill and is in a life-threatening situation on the operating table, it is not unreasonable for the anaesthetist to keep the patient very lightly anaesthetized during this critical phase of the operation. Occasionally, the patient will recall events during the period of light anaesthesia but it is unusual for the patient to sue the anaesthetist, and they are usually very grateful for all the efforts that have been made to save their lives.

Sometimes the patient does not take that attitude and feels that money is needed to compensate for the discomfort of the situation. This would be a case where the Medical Defence Union would fight vigorously on behalf of the anaesthetist because there is no evidence of negligence. Lastly, there is the occasional patient who complains of awareness where the anaesthetic technique appears to be flawless. The complaint would appear to be genuine and the anaesthetic records impeccable, so it is difficult in these cases to know exactly what happened. It could have been a genuine apparatus failure which remained undetected or it could have been that the anaesthetist's records were either not accurate or filled in after the event occurred. The patients in this group only constitute 2.5% of the total number of cases of awareness.

Seniority of anaesthetist

Of all the cases a member of the junior staff was involved in 63% and the remaining 37% were cases anaesthetized by consultants. Many of the junior staff said that they were only carrying out the instructions of their consultants in using a particular technique, and this applied especially to caesarean sections. In some cases a specified technique had been written down and such a document can often be shown to outline a technique that will undoubtedly result in awareness in a proportion of cases. The anaesthetist who has laid down the technique to be followed must bear the blame for errors of the junior staff.

It is distressing to find that more than one-third of cases are the responsibility of anaesthetists of consultant grade, i.e. people with qualifications and experience who should be able to detect signs of awareness in their patients. It may be excusable for a senior house officer in the first 6 months of his job to have a problem with awareness, but there is seldom any reason for a consultant to find himself in the same position.

The claim by the patient

The patient may complain while in hospital, but the first notification that an anaesthetist usually gets is a letter from a solicitor. Later a writ and statement of claim which set out the details of the complaint and the allegations of negligence may be received. Prompt counselling and reassurance by the anaesthetist concerned while the patient is in hospital, and as soon as possible after the event, offer the best chance of avoiding a claim at a later stage. If this fails to work and the anaesthetist receives a solicitor's letter, he should then report the whole matter to his defence society at once. The defence society will refer his case to an anaesthetic adviser, who will be primarily interested in attempting to establish whether or not the claim is genuine. There may be good evidence of awareness, such as a description of the intubation, presence of auditory sensation (in particular details of conversation in the operating theatre), a feeling of paralysis and the inability to communicate with those present in the operating theatre. The patient may also be able to describe the various stages of the operation and the actions of the anaesthetist, perhaps retraction of the eyelids to look at the pupil. Finally, there is often a description of the pain. All this evidence would come from the patient and is not always available in detail when the anaesthetic adviser first assesses the case. It must be accepted that a patient can, in exceptional circumstances, obtain most of his 'evidence' to make a claim from a variety of sources, but in genuine cases some of the facts are difficult to dispute. A genuine claim is usually supported by evidence from the details of the actual anaesthetic, but only when such details are readily available. The absence of anaesthetic records makes defence of a claim, genuine or false, very difficult. A contemporaneous anaesthetic chart is of the greatest value. It may record evidence very suggestive of inadequate anaesthesia. It may display the choice and use of drugs, and the patient's response to them at surgical intervention, in terms of blood pressure, pulse rate and autonomic variables which are not unlikely to be associated with a conscious patient. It is the anaesthetic adviser's task to match the patient's allegations with the anaesthetist's account and the anaesthetic charts. A defence in court can only be made when there is clear evidence against the claim. Lack of such evidence will almost certainly lead a judge to find in favour of the patient. When a claim cannot be defended, or when it appears to be genuine, the defence society concerned will settle the case on behalf of the anaesthetist. If it can be shown that there was a failure in the equipment used by the anaesthetist, and that this failure could not be anticipated or easily detected by the anaesthetist, then the manufacturers of the equipment would be expected to contribute at least in part to the settlement.

Prevention

If we are to prevent an increase in the number of cases of awareness, anaesthetists must be even more meticulous in their techniques. It is not possible to provide a recipe for unconsciousness in every case, but adherence to certain principles will ensure the incidence of awareness is considerably reduced. These principles should include the following:

- A check should be made of all apparatus both in the anaesthetic and the operating rooms before the start of every operating list and, if necessary, before each case.

- Adequate premedication, with perhaps a greater use of amnesic drugs, should be prescribed.
- Proper doses of induction agents should be used. The 'sleep dose' should not be thought of as the upper limit, particularly in fit young individuals. Particular attention should be paid to the dosage of the ultra-short-acting induction agents.
- A volatile agent should be considered for use as part of all these techniques where the patient is to be paralysed and ventilated. Reliance should not be placed on the nitrous oxide:oxygen:narcotic sequence alone as a means to secure unconsciousness.
- When tracheal intubation is difficult, ensure that further doses of induction agent are given when supplements of the relaxant are also given.
- Full reversal of all paralysing drugs should be achieved before the nitrous oxide is turned off. Many patients are aware of the events towards the end of an operation. All patients for a caesarean section should be informed of the possibility of awareness and the reasons behind it. Make sure that such a warning is entered on the anaesthetic record.
- It has been suggested that the use of earplugs on patients would help to cut down the auditory input. This is only acceptable provided all other efforts to prevent awareness are made at the same time.
- All apparatus must be under a service contract and servicing visits made at the correct intervals.

As with all other aspects of anaesthesia, success can only be assured by correct assessment and counselling of patients before operation, the use of equipment which has been shown to be without fault, a meticulous technique and a vigilant attitude throughout the operation and the post-operative period. It is to be hoped that, with this attitude on the part of all anaesthetists, awareness will be eliminated in the future.

Chapter 19

A lawyer's view of the problem

M. J. Powers

Awareness under 'general anaesthesia' – if that is not an oxymoron – occurred long before any aggrieved patient sought to obtain compensation from his luckless anaesthetist. Recent medicolegal interest in this subject in the United Kingdom has been promoted by the widely publicized successful claim brought by Mrs Margaret Ackers in respect of full awareness during a caesarean section which was intended to be under general anaesthesia. This case has led to a flood of similar claims.

The proof of injury

It is a fundamental principle of law that, in order to recover damages from a defendant, the plaintiff must generally establish a definable loss. To have any prospect of success the patient must, therefore, first be able to satisfy the court that he has suffered injury, loss or damage as a consequence of what, without attempting a definition or qualification, can be termed 'inadequate anaesthesia'.

From the patient's point of view, the injury complained of will be physical pain and/or psychological suffering and will be evidenced by the quality and credibility of the patient's own testimony. Supporting medical evidence is essential properly to present the extent of the suffering alleged and to assist in answering the important question: Was it the inadequate anaesthesia which caused the injury complained of?

The problem of causation

The patient who is able to show clearly that an anaesthetist negligently failed to administer adequate anaesthesia will have an easier evidential task proving awareness than where it is more difficult to establish the breach. Until recently, it has been necessary for the plaintiff to prove on the balance of probabilities that the breach of duty/contract caused or materially contributed to injuries alleged (*Bonnington Castings v Wardlaw 1956*). In 1973, in a leading case in the House of Lords on employers' liability, the burden of proof on causation was reversed where the plaintiff was unable to show that the dermatitis injury complained of was caused by the admitted negligence of his employers:

'My Lords, I would suggest that the true view is that, as a rule, when it is proved, on a balance of probabilities, that an employer has been negligent and that his negligence has materially increased the risk of his employee contracting an industrial disease, then he is liable in damages to that employee if he contracts the disease notwithstanding that the employer is not responsible for other factors which have materially contributed to the disease.' Per Lord Salmon *McGhee v National Coal Board* 1973.

Recently, the Court of Appeal considered the position in a case of medical negligence (*Wilsher v Essex Area Health Authority* 1986), and by a majority judgement (the Vice-Chancellor dissenting) eased the plaintiff's difficulty on causation by following the *McGhee* case:

'If it is an established fact that conduct of a particular kind creates a risk that injury will be caused to another or increases an existing risk, injury will ensue; and if the two parties stand in such a relationship that the one party owes a duty not to conduct himself in that way; and if the party does conduct himself in that way; and if the other party does suffer injury of the kind to which the injury related; then the first party is taken to have caused the injury by his breach of duty, even though the existence and extent of the contribution made by the breach cannot be ascertained. If this is the right analysis, it seems to me that the shape taken by the enhancement of the risk ought not be of crucial importance.' Per Mustill LJ in *Wilsher* case.

It would now appear that if the patient is able to show that the nature of her complaints could possibly have been caused by awareness consequent upon inadequate anaesthesia (as opposed, for example, to the normal concomitants of surgery and anaesthesia), she might be relieved of the inherent evidential difficulty of causation and recover damages if it could be shown, on the balance of probabilities, that through the negligence of the anaesthetist, the technique used or the manner in which the anaesthetic was administered and/or monitored, the risk of awareness was materially increased.

Not every injury is compensatable

To determine which established injuries will attract compensation and those which will not, we have to look first at the intention of the anaesthetist and the expectation of his patient. There are situations well recognized by anaesthetists where, without negligence, some pain or discomfort may be felt by the patient undergoing investigation, treatment or surgery not conducted under general anaesthesia. Provided the objectives of analgesia/anaesthesia are properly understood and appreciated by the attendant doctors *and the patient* and the patient's fully informed consent has been obtained, no legal problem arises.

Where the patient's expectations are not achieved, there is always a risk that the patient will seek the lawyer's assistance in the search for incompetence. After all, where the patient without warning remains to some extent aware under intended general anaesthesia, it is not surprising if the question 'Why?' is asked. Explanations *post hoc* rarely satisfy – particularly when they are perfunctory and glib. Such residual confidence as there may have been in the anaesthetist can easily be destroyed by ineptitude in explanation, particularly where there is also a discernible lack of interest in or appreciation of the patient's complaint. It is scarcely surprising that many patients then become interested in determining if the anaesthetist has or has not discharged his obligations (contractual or otherwise) to the requisite standard required of him by the law.

The common duty of care

The author can conceive of no situation in which an anaesthetist could show that no common duty of care was owed to his patient. The real question the anaesthetist has to ask himself is not, 'Do I owe a duty of care?', but 'What is the standard of care required of me?'.

The short answer is that, whatever his training qualification or experience, if he professes an ability to give an anaesthetic he will be required to administer the anaesthetic to the same standard as one would expect from the ordinary skilled and competent anaesthetist. There is no allowance for inexperience or lack of skill (*imperitia culpae annumeratur*). When a learner driver first takes a motor car onto the public road he is required to comply with the standard of the competent qualified driver (*Nettleship v Weston* 1971). If he is unable to achieve such a standard, he will be liable in damages for any consequential injury loss or damage. The same principle applies to the anaesthetist.

'In my view the law requires the trainee or learner to be judged by the same standard as his more experienced colleagues. If it did not, inexperience would frequently be urged as a defence to an action for professional negligence. If this test appears unduly harsh in relation to the inexperienced, I should add that in my view, the inexperienced doctor called upon to exercise a specialist skill will, as part of that skill, seek the advice and help of his superiors when he does or may need it. If he does seek such help, he will in my view often have satisfied the test, even though he may himself have made a mistake.' Per Glidewell LJ in *Wilsher* case.

In respect of diagnosis and treatment (and this may be taken to apply to the administration of anaesthetic), the direction of McNair J to the jury in the case of *Bolam v Friern Hospital Management Committee* 1957 has twice this decade been approved by the House of Lords, first in *Whitehouse v Jordan* 1981 and later in *Maynard v West Midlands Regional Health Authority* 1984.

'. . . I must tell you what in law we mean by 'negligence'. In the ordinary case which does not involve any special skill, negligence in law means a failure to do some act which a reasonable man in the circumstances would do, or the doing of some act which a reasonable man in the circumstances would not do; and if that failure or the doing of that act results in injury, then there is a cause of action. How do you test whether this act or failure is negligent? In the ordinary case it is generally said that you judge it by the action of the man in the street. He is the ordinary man. In one case it has been said you judge by the conduct of the man on the top of the Clapham omnibus. He is the ordinary man. But where you get a situation which involves some special skill or competence, then the test as to whether there has been negligence or not is not the test of the man on the top of the Clapham omnibus, because he has not got that special skill. The test is the standard of the ordinary skilled man exercising and professing to have that special skill. A man need not possess the highest expert skill; it is well established law that it is sufficient if he exercises the ordinary skill of an ordinary competent man exercising that particular art.' Per McNair J in *Bolam* case.

In a later passage, McNair J. cited Lord Clyde, Lord President in *Hunter v Hanley* 1955:

'In the realm of diagnosis and treatment there is ample scope for genuine difference of opinion and one man clearly is not negligent merely because his conclusion differs from that of other professional men, nor because he has displayed less skill or knowledge than others would have shown. The true test for establishing negligence in diagnosis or treatment on the part of a doctor is whether he has been proved to be guilty of such failures that no doctor of ordinary skill would be guilty of if acting with ordinary care.'

The duty to inform

Where, without any failing on the part of the anaesthetist on the foregoing standard in the administration of the anaesthetic, there is a risk of awareness such as may give rise to injury, a patient suffering injury may have an action for breach of the common law duty to inform of the risk of that awareness. Unless there were very good reasons to the contrary (which it would be prudent to record), the anaesthetist would be wise to tell his patient if there were a material risk of awareness, at the same time explaining the reason and offering any necessary reassurance. The majority judgement in the House of Lords in *Sidaway v Bethlem Royal Hospital Governors and others* 1985 imposed in the final analysis a legal duty to inform a patient of certain material risks associated with medical treatment.

'But, even in a case where, as here, no expert witness in the relevant medical field condemns the non-disclosure as being in conflict with responsible and accepted medical practice, I am of the opinion that the judge might in certain circumstances come to the conclusion that the disclosure of a particular risk was so obviously necessary to an informed choice on the part of the patient that no reasonably prudent medical man would fail to make it.' Per Lord Bridge in *Sidaway* case.

Notwithstanding the varying interpretations of their lordships' speeches on the extent of the legal duty to inform, a patient might have a remedy under the *Bolam* test case which was referred to above and in respect of which Lord Diplock in the *Sidaway* case expressed the minority view.

There is probably a duty on an anaesthetist to inform a patient who appears to have been aware under anaesthesia how such awareness came about. In *Lee v South West Thames Regional Health Authority* 1985, the Court of Appeal raised the question as to whether there might be a duty to disclose to a patient after treatment what has in fact been done:

'It should never be forgotten that we are here concerned with a hospital–patient relationship.

The recent decision of the House of Lords in *Sidaway* affirms that a doctor is under a duty to answer his patient's questions as to the treatment proposed. We see no reason why this should not be a similar duty in relation to hospital staff. The duty is subject to the exercise of clinical judgement as to the terms in which the information is given and the extent to which, in the patient's interests, information should be withheld. Why, we ask ourselves, is the position any different if the patient asks what treatment he has in fact had? Let us suppose that a blood transfusion is in contemplation. The patient asks what is involved. He is told that a quantity of blood from a donor will be introduced into his system.

He may ask about the risk of AIDS and so forth and will be entitled to straight answers. He consents. Suppose that, by accident, he is given a quantity of air as well as blood and suffers serious ill effects. Is he not entitled to ask what treatment he in fact received, and is the doctor and hospital authority not obliged to tell him, "in the event you did not only get a blood transfusion. You also got an air transfusion"? Why is the duty different before the treatment from what it is afterwards?

If the duty is the same, then if the patient is refused information to which he is entitled, it must be for consideration whether he could not bring an action for breach of contract claiming specific performance of the duty to inform. In other words, whether the patient could not bring an action for discovery, albeit on a novel basis.

We consider that some thought should be given to what is the duty of disclosure owed by a doctor and a hospital to a patient after treatment, but that is not an issue in this appeal.' Per Sir John Donaldson MR delivering the judgement of the Court.

Private practice – the contractual standard

Where there is a contractual position between the parties the obligations on the anaesthetist may be more exacting. There is an implied term in a contract for medical services that the doctor will exercise reasonable care and skill in the discharge of his duty, and a breach of such a term is actionable *per se*. However, without any injury or loss resulting, such a case would only attract nominal damages and in practice such a case is unlikely to be brought. The standard does not differ from that of the common duty of care unless the anaesthetist expressly warrants that he will provide something more.

'. . . in my opinion, in the absence of any express warranty as to the results of an intended operation, the court should be slow to imply against a medical man an unqualified warranty as to the results of an intended operation, for the very simple reason that, objectively speaking, it is most unlikely that a responsible medical man would intend to give a warranty of this nature. Of course, objectively speaking, it is likely that he would give a guarantee that he would do what he had undertaken to do with reasonable skill and care . . .' Per Slade LJ *Eyre v Measday* 1986.

'. . . I do not consider that a reasonable person would have expected a responsible medical man to be intending to give a guarantee. Medicine, though a highly skilled profession, is not generally regarded as being an exact science. The reasonable man would have expected the defendant to exercise all the proper skill and care of a surgeon in that specialty; he would not in my view have expected the defendant to give a guarantee of 100% success.' Per Neill LJ, *Thake v Maurice* 1986.

These two recent appellate decisions make it clear that there is a presumption against a guarantee in the medical contractual situation. However, if a patient asks the anaesthetist to be sure to put him (the patient) to sleep, the anaesthetist who gives the assurance sought will render himself liable for a breach of the express term should he fail to achieve absence of awareness.

Conclusion

The author has attempted to define the legal problems arising from inadequate anaesthesia, and is firmly of the belief that medicolegal awareness leads to better anaesthetic practice. No professional person should act in a way which he cannot justify and it should be remembered that, in respect of the choice, method of administration and monitoring of anaesthetic, the law leaves the medical profession to judge itself and set its own standards. When injury results· from inadequate anaesthesia, only anaesthetists who are unable to persuade the court that there is a competent body of anaesthetic medical opinion which supports their management of the patient need have any fear of being found negligent.

There is an enormous range of anaesthetic techniques considered acceptable by the profession. There are some techniques, however, that are no longer acceptable or justifiable. Regrettably, fear of compromising professional freedom seems to be the principal reason for the failure of the professional anaesthetic bodies to establish and publish criteria of acceptable practice. It is to be hoped that this book will in some measure fill that void and serve as both illumination and guidance to all anaesthetists wishing to serve the best interests of their patients rather than their lawyers.

Table of cases

Bolam v Friern Hospital Management Committee [1957] 1 WLR 582
Bonnington Castings v Wardlaw [1956] AC 613
Eyre v Measday [1986] 1 All ER 488, CA
Hunter v Hanley (1955) SLT 213
Lee v South West Thames Regional Health Authority [1985] 2 All ER 385
McGhee v National Coal Board [1973] 1 WLR 1, HL
Maynard v West Midlands Regional Health Authority [1984] 1 WLR 634
Nettleship v Weston [1971] 2 QB 691
Sidaway v Bethlem Royal Hospital Governors and others [1985] 1 All ER 643
Thake v Maurice [1986] 1 All ER 497, CA
Whitehouse v Jordan [1981] 1 WLR 246
Wilsher v Essex Area Health Authority [1986] 3 ALL ER 801

Chapter 20

Awareness under anaesthesia: a QC's view

M. Puxon

It is indicative of the present sensitive state of the medical profession that a gathering of experts should spend considerable time and energy in examining the possibility of complaints being made by patients that they were inadequately, although not dangerously, anaesthetized. It is also a credit to the profession. It is extraordinary that, with the increase in claims in medical negligence, it was not until June 1985 that such a claim reached the courts and was reported. The author knows from personal experience that other cases were started and settled, and indeed one was heard (unreported), but the plaintiff was unsuccessful in establishing negligence against the anaesthetist.

It is clear from Chapter 18 that a number of claims have followed the 1985 successful case *Ackers v Wigan Health Authority*, and that a number of these claims are genuine enough and will have been settled by the defence societies. But a larger number of the complaints made since 1985 are ill-founded; that is not to say that the patient is not genuine in the belief that there was awareness, but such belief can be engendered by the knowledge of other claims, supported by the fantasies which are likely to accompany the drugged state and the nervous shock accompanying any major operative procedure. The increasing number of genuine claims, although small, may well indicate the reluctance of the medical profession as a whole to over-anaesthetize, and the consciousness that all administrations of drugs have dangers and that dosage should be well on the side of safety. This must be particularly so in the case of obstetric anaesthesia, where there are two patients to be considered, and the administration of potentially harmful inhalation and intravenous drugs is a special threat to the child.

The *Ackers* case referred to in *Current Law*, March 1986, was a clear case of a failure by an anaesthetist to ensure that the patient was not only paralysed, but unaware and unable to feel: she was conscious of everything that was done to her and suffered greatly. It was an undoubted case of negligence and the only dispute was as to the quantum of damages. What is chiefly of interest here, however, is not the case where sensation remains at 100%, but where the patient, while feeling no pain, is yet aware of what is going on in the operating theatre and is thereby distressed and consequently suffers some upset after the operation. Such cases are unlikely to give rise to a large claim in damages, and most can be settled out of court, but it is important that anaesthetists should realize what can be made the proper basis of a claim in negligence, and how they can avoid such claims, or even an initial complaint.

There follow a few comments, some from the author's own experience, and some views on how the present state of the law applies in this field.

Consent: how much information is required?

It is difficult to see how 'informed consent' in the North American sense can be obtained in anaesthetic cases. Happily, as the courts have said, there is no place for the full doctrine of 'informed' consent in English Law; what is required is that the patient should give consent to any procedure with a knowledge of 'any dangers which are special in kind or magnitude or special to the patient' (Lord Templeman in *Sidaway v Bethlem Royal Hospital Governors and others* 1985). This does not include telling the patient of every risk which may properly be said to accompany the procedure; for example, patients are not told that a certain percentage of general anaesthetics end in cardiac arrest and even, although very rarely nowadays, in death. Should a patient be warned that the administration of a general anaesthetic may leave him or her aware of what is going on? Or even sensible to the pain of the operative procedures? As Lord Templeman said in the *Sidaway* case:

> The doctor must decide in the light of his training and experience and in the light of his knowledge of the patient what should be said and how it should be said . . . . . . At the end of the day, the doctor, bearing in mind the best interests of the patient and bearing in mind the patient's right to information which will enable the patient to make a balanced judgment, must decide what information should be given to the patient and in what terms that information should be couched'.

At another part of his judgment Lord Templeman said:

> 'The provision of too much information may prejudice the attainment of the objective of restoring the patient's health.'

To warn that there is a risk of awareness, whether of pain or surrounding events, would upset most patients to a degree which must be to their disadvantage, and it cannot therefore be seen that the question of consent can ever be of relevance in these cases. It certainly provides a fertile field for difficulty and heartsearching in obstetrics where consent to an epidural is being considered, and the patient is unfit to give any real consent, but that is a different problem.

The risk/benefit consideration

It cannot be too strongly emphasized that for any plaintiff to succeed in establishing negligence, whether against a doctor or anybody else, he or she must prove, on the balance of probabilities, that what was done amounted to a breach of care owed by the defendant (*see* Chapter 19). If, therefore, the defendant can satisfy the court that what he did was for the benefit of the patient, and that he carried out the procedure with the skill and care required of a medical man exercising his speciality, the plaintiff will not succeed. If there exists a body of professional opinion, which is competent and supports the methods used by the doctor and the decisions reached by him at the time of the procedure, then the court will hold that the defendant was not negligent. If, for example, an anaesthetist were to decide on a particular method of anaesthesia which carried extra risks of awareness, but was, he believed, necessary for the safety and health of the patient, and if that cause were supported by a body of competent professional opinion, the fact that the patient suffered as a result would not lead to a finding of negligence. Such a situation would arise only rarely: it is used as an example of the risk/benefit equation which the courts have to consider. In this respect the author would refer to *Maynard v West Midlands Regional Health Authority* 1985, where the House of Lords stressed that the court may not choose between one respectable body of professional opinion and another; if there is *any* 'body of competent professional opinion' which supports the actions of the defendant, the fact that there is *another* 'body of competent professional opinion' which holds a different view would not assist the plaintiff. The burden of proof remains upon the plaintiff and, if there is this element of conflict between authorities in the speciality, the plaintiff will not succeed. The burden of proof remains throughout upon the plaintiff. The only exception to this rule is where the injury suffered can only be explained, *prima facie*, by the negligence of the doctor (*res ipsa loquitur*); the burden of proof then shifts, and the doctor must show that there was no negligence.

It has to be accepted that the purpose of general anaesthesia is to remove sensation, both of pain and of general awareness. It is difficult to envisage a case where a patient would not succeed in showing a degree of negligence if both aware and sensitive to pain during general anaesthesia, save in the circumstances referred to in Chapter 18.

Avoidance of complaint

But it is not the rare case which reaches the stage of proceedings being launched that is the real worry to the anaesthetist. As a responsible professional man, his anxiety is that his patient should not suffer, and should not be in a position to complain. The anaesthetist will never be able to avoid the truly spurious claims: those should be weeded out very quickly, especially if the precautions mentioned by Hargrove (Chapter 18) and Powers (Chapter 19) are taken up. But what of the cases where the patient genuinely believes that he or she has cause for complaint when nothing has gone wrong with the anaesthetic? It is the author's belief that the majority of such cases could be nipped in the bud by proper communication. As in other branches of the art, doctors and patients do not always understand each other, and the doctors and nurses may generate a feeling of lack of confidence by unwillingness or inability to explain the irrational reactions of their patients. Every complaint should be listened to with care and sympathy; where the complaint smacks of the truth, a full investigation should be carried out, and where appropriate due apology given. Where the complaint is based on some degree of fantasy, a full explanation of the effects of surgery and anaesthesia and the drugs administered may well satisfy the patient that there is no basis for complaint and that in any event no harm has been done. The longer such doubts and anxieties are allowed to fester in the patient's mind, the greater the difficulty in removing them and the greater the injury likely to be done. In these cases time expended with the patient at an early stage is well spent.

Finally, some words of comfort from Lord Scarman in the *Sidaway* case:

'The law . . . operates not in Utopia, but in the world as it is.'

It is reassuring to know that the highest court in the land approaches questions of medical negligence in such a practical way.

Table of cases

Ackers v Wigan Health Authority (1985) referred to in Current Law, March 1986
Maynard v West Midlands Regional Health Authority [1985] 1 All ER 635
Sidaway v Bethlem Royal Hospital Governors and others [1985] 1 All ER 6

Chapter 21

An American legal view

B. H. Thompson

The possibility that a patient might be conscious and aware of an operation despite being under general anaesthesia has not caught the attention of the American legal system as it has of the British. Although suits alleging that a patient was conscious during an operation are not unheard of in the USA, the writer has found no reported instance of a plaintiff prevailing on such an allegation. Perhaps, for this reason, there do not appear to be as many claims brought in the USA for 'consciousness under anaesthesia', as earlier chapters have suggested the UK is currently seeing.

The author has only been able to find one reported lawsuit in the USA that directly involved consciousness under anaesthesia. In *Turner v Malone* 1985, a plaintiff who had undergone an operation to remove a malignancy in his lung sued the anaesthesiologist for medical malpractice and alleged that he was conscious during much of the operation. The patient's description of this experience parallels those discussed in other chapters, except that the patient alleged he was able not only to hear and to feel pain but also to see some of what was going on:

> 'Turner [the plaintiff] was given preparatory anesthetic injections prior to being brought to the operating room which caused great drowsiness but did not completely anesthetize him. After arrival in the operating arena, he was further given anesthesia by Dr. Malone, a registered anesthesiologist. The additional anesthesia rendered Turner physically immobile (i.e., partially paralyzed) but did not wholly cause him to be amnestic. Thus, Turner could observe what the surgeons were doing and saying but could not speak, blink his eyes, or otherwise move. He observed the surgeon pick up something shiny and felt intense pain when the surgeon made apparently what was a surgical opening of the chest cavity. He further felt great pressure apparently when a rib separator was applied to open the rib cage in order to allow the surgeon to reach the lung. At this point, Turner passed into unconsciousness and experienced no further operative pain.'
> *Turner* case.

The jury returned a verdict in favour of the anaesthesiologist after hearing all of the evidence and, because it was a jury trial, we do not know the reasoning behind the verdict.

One other published case involved tangential allegations of consciousness under anaesthesia. In *Aubert v Charity Hosp* 1978, the plaintiff alleged that his wife died following childbirth by caesarean section because of errors on the part of the anaesthesiologist. According to the plaintiff, the anaesthesiologist inserted a tracheal tube into the patient's oesophagus, rather than her trachea, and failed to discover the mistake in time, resulting in hypoxia, irreversible brain damage, and ultimately death (*Aubert* case). As part of his lawsuit, the plaintiff sought damages for pain and suffering to his wife on the theory that 'after the initial anesthesia (two minutes of cyclopropane) wore off, the continuing anesthesia (ethylene) did not take effect because the tube was improperly placed' (*Aubert* case). The court, however, refused to award any damages for pain and suffering on the grounds that the evidence of consciousness and pain was simply too speculative.

Other sources of information on anaesthesia malpractice confirm that there have been few lawsuits in the USA alleging consciousness under anaesthesia. Anaesthesiologists have been a frequent target of malpractice suits in the USA[1], but these suits have focused primarily on overdoses of anaesthetic drugs, problems in tracheal intubation, complications in spinal anaesthesia, and other incidents of negligence leading to physical injury or death. In a recent study of over 100 insurance files claiming anaesthesia malpractice, none of the claims involved consciousness under anaesthesia[2]. Seminars and treatises on the legal aspects of anaesthesia do not even note the possibility of consciousness under anaesthesia[3,4].

In spite of the paucity of such suits, however, it is worth considering the major types of legal claims that might arise when a patient is conscious during an operation despite being under anaesthesia. There is no obvious reason why suits alleging consciousness under anaesthesia should be more common in the UK than in the USA; and the relative notoriety of *Ackers v Wigan Health Authority* (1985) may lead to more allegations of consciousness under anaesthesia in the USA, just as it has in the UK.

Malpractice claims

A patient who sues because he or she was allegedly conscious during an operation is most likely to sue for medical malpractice. As in the UK, such a patient will have to overcome a variety of hurdles. To begin with, the patient will have to convince the decision maker, whether jury or judge, that he or she was indeed conscious during the operation. In some cases, this should be easy: when, for example, the plaintiff can give a detailed description of the operation or the doctors' conversation during the operation. But in many cases where such ready corroboration is not present, the decision maker may well find the plaintiff's claim far too speculative to support an award.

Next the plaintiff will have to show that he or she was conscious because of the anaesthesiologist's negligence. As in the UK, an anaesthesiologist in the USA does not, apart from some special contractual agreement, ensure that the patient will be unconscious and feel no pain. To prevail, a plaintiff will have to show not only that the anaesthesiologist did not exercise that degree of skill, care, knowledge, or attention ordinarily exercised by other anaesthesiologists in similar situations*, but also that the plaintiff was conscious *because* of this deficiency.

---

*The exact standard of skill or care to which the anaesthesiologist will be held will vary from jurisdiction to jurisdiction within the USA. In some jurisdictions, for example, the defendant-anaesthesiologist will be compared with anaesthesiologists within the same locality; in other jurisdictions, the comparison will be with anaesthesiologists nationally.

If the plaintiff can show that the anaesthesiologist did not exercise reasonable skill or care in a way that heightened the chances of consciousness, the plaintiff will probably find it relatively easy to show causation. The trick will be proving the first element. It will not be enough to show that some, or even a majority of, anaesthesiologists would have done things differently from the defendant. So long as the defendant chose and administered the anaesthetics in a manner acceptable to a respected segment of anaesthesiologists, the defendant will generally prevail (*see*, for example, *Chumbler v McClure* 1974 and *Furey v Thomas Jefferson Univ Hosp* 1984). The plaintiff, in short, will have the heavy burden of showing through *expert* testimony that the defendant did not administer anaesthetics in a reasonable fashion.

In most American jurisdictions, the plaintiff can try to overcome this burden by arguing that the doctrine of *res ipsa loquitur* should apply. If the plaintiff can show that a patient will not ordinarily be conscious under anaesthesia unless the anaesthesiologist were negligent, the burden will switch to the defendant to prove that he was not negligent*. The medical chapters of this book, however, suggest that the plaintiff will find it difficult to prove the predicate for *res ipsa loquitur*. Courts are particularly reticent to apply *res ipsa loquitur* to disputes over the choice of medical treatments or techniques – to a choice, for example, between using light levels of anaesthesia with a risk of consciousness and using deeper levels of anaesthesia with their alternative dangers[5].

Even if the plaintiff establishes medical malpractice, the plaintiff may find it difficult to recover damages in some states. In a few states, for example, a plaintiff cannot collect damages for emotional distress in the absence of some physical injury (*see Holler v United States* 1983; Restatement 2d Torts § 436A). If a patient was conscious during an operation but felt no pain, the patient arguably is not entitled to any damages in such a state (although the courts will probably try hard to find a theory upon which to award damages).

Contract claims

Even if the anaesthesiologist was not negligent, a patient may still have a viable law suit against the doctor if the anaesthesiologist was careless enough to warrant that the patient would not be conscious during the operation. In most American jurisdictions, a patient can sue for breach of contract if his or her doctor has broken an express promise to the patient even though the breach is not the result of malpractice (*see Scarzella v Saxon* 1981).

Anaesthesiologists (along with medical personnel involved in an operation) should, therefore, be very careful in what they say to patients before an operation. Some states permit suits for breach of contract only where the contract is in writing (*see*, for example, Ariz. Rev. Stat. § 12-562(c)). In most states, however, doctors should avoid the temptation to calm a patient by telling him or her that 'There's nothing to this operation' or 'You'll feel nothing', lest a court later conclude that

---

*See, for example, *Carnacchia v Mount Vernon Hosp* 1983 (applying *res ipsa loquitur* where tracheal intubation led to the patient's dentures becoming lodged in his oesophagus). In order to get a court to apply *res ipsa loquitur*, a plaintiff must also show that the defendant had exclusive control of the instruments that led to the defendant's injury and that the plaintiff could not have contributed to the injury. Both of these requirements would generally be met in a case of consciousness under anaesthesia.

the doctor warranted that the patient would not be conscious or feel any pain during the operation. While some courts will recognize such statements as pure puffery not intended to warrant anaesthetic results, other courts may well conclude that the doctor did guarantee the results*.

Informed consent claims

Anaesthesiologists in the USA must be concerned, not only with what they say to a patient before an operation, but also with what they do not say. Unless a patient has been told ahead of time that there is a risk that he or she may be conscious during part of an operation, the patient who ends up listening to the operation or feeling pain may well sue the anaesthesiologist on the ground that he or she did not give informed consent to such an unusual opportunity.

When an anaesthesiologist believes that there is a recognizable risk that a patient may find himself or herself conscious during an operation, the safest legal course of action is to tell the patient of the possibility. Such a warning is the only sure way of guaranteeing that the patient will not sue for lack of informed consent (or at least will not win).

The anaesthesiologist may decide in particular settings, however, that a warning is not in the patient's best interest: that a warning could create physiological reactions that would increase the risks of the operation or could lead the patient to reject the safest anaesthetic technique for purely irrational reasons; or the anaesthesiologist may find it impractical to tell the patient of the risk because of the emergency nature of the operation. What risks does the anaesthesiologist run in not warning the patient in such circumstances?

The courts generally recognize that there are situations like these where disclosure of risks would be either unwise or useless. But the American law of informed consent varies dramatically from state to state and belies easy answers. For that reason, it is worth briefly considering the various issues that are likely to arise in any lawsuit in which the plaintiff alleges that he or she was not informed of the risk of being conscious under anaesthesia.

The major issue will be whether the anaesthesiologist had any duty to inform the patient of the risk of being conscious. In most states, that issue will initially boil down to typical anaesthesiologist practice; would a reasonable anaesthesiologist have warned the patient of the risk?† In a number of states, however, the issue will focus on what the patient would have wanted to know in order to protect his or her interests: would the risk of being conscious be something that an average, reasonable patient would have considered material in deciding whether to undergo the operation as planned?‡

---

*Compare *McKinney v Nash* 1981 (comment that surgery would be 'simple and without problem' was not a contractual warranty) with *Guilmet v Campbell* 1971 (affirming jury finding that statements that the operation 'takes care of all your troubles' and 'there is no danger at all' were warranties).

†*See*, for example, *Karp v Cooley* 1974. Here, as in basic malpractice, states differ in whether they look to the practice of other local anaesthesiologists or to anaesthesiologists nationwide.

‡*See*, for example, *Canterbury v Spence* 1972. In some states, the question is whether the *plaintiff*, not a hypothetical 'reasonable plaintiff', would have considered the information material. *See*, for example, *Scott v Bradford* 1979.

As a practical matter, the courts in these latter states will weigh two factors in deciding whether the anaesthesiologist should have warned the patient of the risk of being conscious: the statistical chance that the patient would find himself or herself aware of the operation despite being anaesthetized, and the court's perception of how traumatic a patient would find being aware of the operation while anaesthetized. A court will generally be more willing to agree with the doctor's decision not to warn where a risk was extremely remote and the consequences not particularly dire, for example, than when the risk was significant and the consequences severe.

Here, the medical chapters in this book (along with common sense) suggest that being conscious but paralysed during a major operation can be a severely traumatic event (although steps can be taken to reduce the trauma). Thus, the major issue will probably be how much risk there is of being conscious in a particular setting. If the risk is only one in 10 000, the courts are unlikely to find the anaesthesiologist liable; if the risk is, say, 5%, on the other hand, the doctor runs considerably more danger if he fails to inform the patient of the risk.

Even if the courts conclude that the information is of the type that should normally be revealed to a patient, they might recognize that there may be situations in which the doctor may reasonably decide not to tell a particular patient for valid medical reasons. Under the so-called 'therapeutic privilege', an anaesthesiologist will generally not be liable for failing to tell a patient of the risks of being conscious if the patient's emotional state was fragile enough that telling the patient ran the risk of making the operation more dangerous or leading the patient irrationally to reject the safest anaesthetic technique (*see*, for example, *Nishi v Hartwell* 1970 and *Roberts v Woods* 1962).

The courts also recognize that disclosure of risks is not always practical during emergencies[5]. Where a patient is unconscious or otherwise incapable of consent, but an immediate operation is necessary, the anaesthesiologist will not be faulted for failing to disclose to the patient that he or she may be conscious during the operation. The courts, however, apply this exception very narrowly (*see*, for example, *Gravis v Physicians & Surgeons Hosp* 1968).

Even if the patient can convince the court that he or she should have been warned of the risk, the anaesthesiologist has not yet lost. The patient must still show that, if warned, he or she would have insisted on a different anaesthetic technique or foregone the operation entirely (*see*, for example, *Cobbs v Grant* 1972). The patient may find this difficult to prove where the anaesthetic technique followed was the least risky course. Most patients would prefer to be conscious than dead.

Conclusion

No matter what the law, the most important thing to the anaesthesiologist is to avoid being dragged into court in the first place. Even if you ultimately win, it is a depressing experience to be served with a complaint and to have to suffer the inconveniences of the modern lawsuit. And no matter how strong your case, it is not always easy to get a court to dismiss a lawsuit at an early stage.

Perhaps the best way in which anaesthesiologists can attempt to stay out of court is to increase their rapport and contact with their patients. Except when there is a valid reason not to, the anaesthesiologist should make sure patients are aware of any significant risk of consciousness under anaesthesia. When an anaesthesiologist believes during and operation that a patient may be conscious, the anaesthesiologist should take steps to make the experience easier on the patient, for example, by talking to the patient during the operation and reassuring the patient. When there is any indication after an operation that a patient may have been conscious, the anaesthesiologist should sit down with the patient and talk to him or her about what happened. The anaesthesiologist should sympathize with and respond to any concerns of the patient and make sure that the patient receives any necessary therapy. A lawsuit is most likely to arise when communications between the anaesthesiologist and the patient break down.

References

1. NATIONAL ASSOCIATION OF INSURANCE COMMISSIONERS (1980) *Malpractice Claims: Final Compilation*, pp. 164–168
2. ECKENHOFF (1984) *Observations Drawn from a Review of 104 Anesthesia Malpractice Suits*. Paper delivered at Illinois Society of Anesthesiologists, 11th April
3. DORNETTE, W. H. L. (Ed.) (1972) *Legal Aspects of Anesthesia*. Philadelphia: F. A. Davis
4. WASMUTH, C. E. (1961) *Anesthesia and the Law*. Springfield, Illinois: C. C. Thomas
5. LOUISELL, D. and WILLIAMS, H. (1983) *Medical Malpractice,* paragraph 14.04 at 14-56 and paragraph 22.04 at 22-10. New York: Mathew Bender

Table of cases

Ackers v Wigan Health Authority (1985) *see* Chapter 20
Aubert v Charity Hosp. of La, 363 So. 2d 1223 (La. App. 1978)
Cantberbury v Spence, 464 F. 2d 772, 786–788 (D.C. Cir.), *cert. denied*, 409 U.S. 1064 (1972)
Carnacchia v Mount Vernon Hosp., 93 App. Div. 2d 851, 461 N.Y.S. 2d 348 (1983)
Chumbler v McClure, 505 F. 2d 489, 492 (6th Cir. 1974)
Cobbs v Grant, 8 Cal. 3d 229, 104 Cal. Rptr. 505, 502 P. 2d 1, 11–12 (1972)
Furey v Thomas Jefferson Univ. Hosp., 325 Pa. Super. 212, 472 A. 2d 1083, 1089–91 (1984)
Gravis v Physicians & Surgeons Hosp., 427 S.W. 2d 310 (Tex. 1968)
Guilmet v Campbell, 385 Mich. 57, 188 N.W. 2d 601 (1971)
Holler v United States, 724 F. 2d 104 (10th Cir. 1983)
Karp v Cooley, 493 F. 2d 408, 419–420 (5th Cir.), *cert. denied*, 419 U.S. 845 (1974)
McKinney v Nash, 120 Cal. App. 3d 428, 174 Cal. Rptr. 642 (3rd Dist. 1981)
Nishi v Hartwell, 52 Haw. 188 & 296, 473 P. 2d 116, 119–121 (1970)
Roberts v Woods, 206 F. Supp. 579, 583 (S.D. Ala. 1962)
Scarzella v Saxon, 436 A. 2d 358 (D.C. 1981)
Scott v Bradford, 606 P. 2d 554, 558–559 (Okla. 1979)
Turner v Malone, 176 Ga. App. 132, 335, S.E. 2d 404 (1985)

Chapter 22

Awareness: Clinical aspects

J. E. Utting

The paradoxical term 'awareness during general anaesthesia' invites a debate which would involve philosophers and psychologists as well as anaesthetists. The gordian knot must be cut or paralysis will result. In this chapter, therefore, the term 'awareness during general anaesthesia' will be used to describe the phenomenon in which the patient is able to recall events which occurred when he or she was thought to be completely unaware of anything because of the influence of anaesthetic agents.

This, it will readily be realized, is a dangerously simplistic definition, as some other contributions to this book show; at the simplest level we can say that we can forget what we have experienced. Taking this argument to its extremes, it might be suggested that patients do know everything which goes on when they are supposed to be under the influence of a general anaesthetic, but that this is not brought to consciousness since they are unable to recall it.

This seems fundamentally unlikely. There are over three million anaesthetics given each year in the United Kingdom and many of the patients having these anaesthetics have had one or more anaesthetics previously. If they had been aware of what went on during previous anaesthetics, it would be expected that they would approach subsequent anaesthesia with marked apprehension amounting to terror.

There is no doubt that most patients remain apprehensive about anaesthesia, even when they have had a previous anaesthetic, but those who have already jumped by parachute still feel anxious when the next jump comes: there are features of both activities which invite anxiety. This is in sharp contrast to many of those who do claim to have been overtly aware during anaesthesia; they often (though not always) approach further anaesthesia with a specific and real fear – the fear that they may be aware again.

The account which follows is based almost entirely on asking patients about what they remember. This immediately raises the obvious objection that a patient may remember today and forget tomorrow and (surprisingly) vice versa. The question as to when the questions should be asked appears to be critical.

This difficulty, however, may be more apparent than real. Once the patient has fully recovered from anaesthesia it probably matters little when, within, say, the first 3 days, he or she is asked questions about his or her experiences, for, though what is trivial may be readily forgotten, awareness of surgery and very unpleasant dreams will be remembered. This is really a statement which could be summarized by saying that what is memorable is remembered, at least in the short term. From the point of view of litigation, the importance of this is obvious.

Historical aspects

George Crile described a case of consciousness under anaesthesia with nitrous oxide occurring in 1908[1], when the patient was breathing spontaneously. However, awareness during general anaesthesia when the patient is not paralysed with muscle relaxant drugs and, therefore, able to move in response to nociceptive stimuli is probably too rare an event to need further discussion. It was after the introduction of the muscle relaxants that awareness under anaesthesia first became a clinical problem of importance, for here the situation is that the patient may be conscious but unable to move because he or she is paralysed and respiration is controlled.

The first case of this sort was reported by Winterbottom[2]. Here there was technical error; both the nitrous oxide and cyclopropane supply ran out at the same time; both were being used to keep the patient anaesthetized. Since then there have been a large number of case reports, studies, reviews and editorials on the subject. The first systematic investigation into the subject was by Hutchinson[3] and the whole subject has recently been reviewed[4].

It is not now commonly remembered that the introduction of the muscle relaxants into anaesthesia was initially a disaster in some parts of the world. The reason was that the agents were being used as auxiliary agents to pre-existing techniques, when a new and radical approach was required. For example, it is possible, though difficult, to perform a partial gastrectomy with diethyl ether as the sole anaesthetic agent. But simply to add a non-depolarizing muscle relaxant to the technique without in any other way modifying it is dangerous; for example, respiratory depression may be fatal during or after surgery.

It is not surprising, therefore, that Beecher and Todd in 1954 found, in a large survey of anaesthesia in teaching institutions in the USA, that the use of the relaxant drugs was dangerous, being associated with a high mortality[5]. From this the erroneous conclusion was made that the muscle relaxants were intrinsically unsafe – a conclusion to which many others had come independently.

The method which subsequently became known, mainly in the USA, as the Liverpool technique had been established by using the muscle relaxants as new agents and radically adapting anaesthetic practice to meet what was essentially a new situation[6,7]. From this arose the concept of anaesthesia as a 'tetrad' (of narcosis, reflex suppression, muscular relaxation and controlled ventilation) with specific drugs used to subserve specific purposes. Reversal of the residual action of the non-depolarizing agent was regarded as mandatory.

Nitrous oxide, often combined with 'heavy' premedication, was used as the sole anaesthetic agent. At the time in which the technique was introduced, the only other gaseous and volatile agents were limited in number and quality – for example, ether, cyclopropane, chloroform and the like. Nor was it possible to administer the volatile agents with any accuracy; even after the discovery of halothane a temperature-compensated vaporizer was not generally available for some time. It was against this background that the use of nitrous oxide as the sole agent came to be widely accepted.

Clinical features of awareness

With the most complete failure of anaesthesia, the patient knows where he or she (usually the latter) is (i.e. in the operating theatre), knows what is happening (i.e.

that she is being operated on), hears conversation, feels pain, knows that she is paralysed and would like to signal her predicament but is unable to do so. It is relatively uncommon for the patient to recall seeing anything, but this does happen. The episode of consciousness may last from a few seconds to an hour or more.

There is, more frequently, an incomplete picture, for example, the patient may hear conversation and may realize what is going on but may feel no pain. Sometimes there may be considerable difficulty in deciding if the patient really was awake or not, and even the patient may not be sure. Awareness is usually, though surprisingly not invariably, considered by the patient to be an horrific experience.

A woman of 29 was presented for stripping of bilateral varicose veins: she was fit and took neither drugs nor alcohol. After surgery she claimed to have been awake during anaesthesia for dental extractions on two occasions. Her account was quite compatible with what went on in the operating theatre. 'When I woke up I was lying flat. I knew I was in the operating theatre, though I couldn't see anything; it was as though I was in a cave. I couldn't move a muscle and I felt someone lift up my leg. I heard Mr X say "I'll paint this side, but you can paint the other". Then he asked the anaesthetist if he'd been to the medical board last night and he said he hadn't. Mr X told the anaesthetist about some of the things which went on at the meeting. I thought, O God, they're going to cut me and they don't know that I'm awake. I could feel tears in my eyes and I tried to keep them coming. I thought they would be bound to know I was awake if they saw I was crying. Then Mr X said "How about a knife, sister?" I thought "This is it!" and I felt a terrible pain in my groin. Then I must have blacked out.' It might be added that the patient's description of the conversation was entirely accurate (there was a tape-recorder running at the time) and that alone among 500 records were recorded, at the beginning of the anaesthetic, the words 'lacrimating +++'.

Sequelae of awareness

Patients who have been subjected to this experience frequently develop a traumatic neurosis[8-10]. They show clinical features of both anxiety and depression; they have recurrent nightmares in which they may re-live their experiences; they are afraid to go to sleep because they fear the nightmares or fear that they may die before they wake up; when they do wake up they may find themselves frantically trying to puzzle out whether they are alive or dead. There is often a reluctance to talk to anyone because it may be thought that they are mad. Symptoms may last for a year or more and may be accompanied by varying degrees of anxiety and/or depression. They may be discernibly psychiatrically ill.

Such patients may respond to a sympathetic hearing and to a careful explanation of what has happened. In cases of doubt, however, psychiatric assistance should be sought.

If, in the post-operative period, the patient should complain of awareness (or if such a complaint be accidentally elicited), the patient should be sympathetically interviewed by an anaesthetist – preferably a senior anaesthetist. Denying that the patient was aware when she undoubtedly was is unethical; not only is it mendacious in itself, but it may be harmful to the patient, making the patient doubt his or her own sanity.

Dreaming

When light anaesthesia is used, the patient may recall dreams that appeared to be associated with the anaesthetic[11]. Most dreams are probably forgotten and most of those which are remembered 24 hours after surgery are pleasant, not infrequently involving situations in which alcohol figures.

These dreams, however, are sometimes unpleasant; occasionally they may appear to be dictated by the operation – for example, a woman having a repair of uterovaginal prolapse dreamed that she was having a baby. But the most unpleasant dreams are on themes which might be described, in broad terms, as transcendental: the mystery of the universe has been revealed and it is purely evil, the world has been taken over by the Devil, and so on. These dreams can be very disturbing; indeed, sometimes they can lead to the syndrome of traumatic neurosis which has already been mentioned.

There is no absolute proof that dreaming reported to an interviewer say 24 hours after anaesthesia actually took place while the patient was anaesthetized; it might, for example, have happened in the recovery room. Nevertheless, there are indications that dreaming does occur during light anaesthesia. It is tempting to assume that there is a continuum, that adequate anaesthesia results in a patient's complete inability to recall anything, that a lighter anaesthesia may result in remembered dreams and that a still lighter (and inadequate) anaesthetic will result in the patient's being aware. This assumption could, of course, only be valid if the depth of anaesthesia were constant.

Even when nitrous oxide is used alone with muscle relaxants, the incidence of awareness during anaesthesia is low and it is difficult, therefore, to assess the effects of different techniques on this incidence; the incidence of dreaming, however, is much higher and is reduced readily by, for example, using the volatile agents as adjuvants. From this it is tempting to assume that the use of such adjuvants is likely to reduce the incidence of awareness.

Nitrous oxide as the sole anaesthetic

The best way to test the problems of awareness and dreaming in association with anaesthesia with muscle relaxant is to use nitrous oxide alone. *Table 22.1* shows the results from an investigation of this type of technique.

Table 22.1 Results of questioning patients after anaesthesia with two techniques: relaxant with nitrous oxide as the sole anaesthetic agent and nitrous oxide supplemented with halothane 0.5%

Number of patients	N_2O/O_2 only	N_2O/O_2/halothane
Total number	500	100
Certainly aware	2 (0.4%) ⎱ 2.2%	0
Possibly aware	9 (1.8%) ⎰	0
Dreams worst feature of surgery	35* (7.0%)	2 (2%)

* Includes 12 out of 13 patients in whom dreams were suggested by surgery.

The 500 patients included were presented for a wide variety of general surgical procedures. They were aged 17–80 years and weighed between 32 and 100 kg; there was a preponderance of women (323) over men (267). In theatre, anaesthesia was given by one of six anaesthetists and was monitored by another anaesthetist using an oxygen analyser and (later) a tape-recorder to give a record of what was said. If it was deemed that there was a technical error in the anaesthetic, the patient was excluded from the trial. The patients were interviewed by one of five anaesthetists or by one of two clinical psychologists. These interviews were conducted between 18 and 36 hours after surgery.

The method of anaesthesia was stereotyped. Premedication was with promethazine 25–50 mg orally the night before surgery. Induction of anaesthesia was with thiopentone 100–350 mg given rapidly and either preceded or followed by tubocurarine 30–45 mg. The patient breathed nitrous oxide (70%) in oxygen (30%) almost immediately after this and positive pressure ventilation of the lungs with the mixture was established as soon as possible. Tracheal intubation was effected 2–5 minutes after the relaxant had been administered. Positive pressure ventilation was re-established using the same mixture as before, and ventilation continued by hand or using a ventilator which had previously been 'run through' with nitrous oxide and oxygen. No volatile adjuvant or narcotic supplement was used.

Increments of tubocurarine were given when clinically indicated. At the end of surgery, atropine 1.2 mg and neostigmine 5.0 mg were administered. When spontaneous ventilation had been established, the patient was allowed to breathe oxygen for about a minute before the tracheal tube was removed.

Of the 500 patients, two (0.4%) were certainly aware: one was the patient described in the case history earlier; she developed most of the symptoms of traumatic neurosis. The other, a man of 55 who was having a gastro-enterostomy and vagotomy, was able to relate two snatches of conversation; he knew what was happening but felt no pain and was none the worse, it would seem, for his experience.

A further nine patients (1.8%) were possibly aware, but neither they nor the investigators were sure. The period of awareness, if there was awareness, was very short. The total incidence was, therefore, 2.2%. A much larger percentage of the patients (7%), however, had dreams which they thought were the worst feature of their visit to the operating theatre – worse even than pre-operative anxiety and post-operative pain.

The incidence of awareness found in this study is not dissimilar to that found in obstetric practice. Thus, when nitrous oxide (67%) is used in obstetrics, the incidence of awareness is between 2.5 and 4% – when a 50% mixture was used up to 25% of the mothers were aware[12].

Adjuvants to nitrous oxide

Premedication

There is not a great deal of information available on the influence of premedication on the incidence of awareness and/or dreaming, and some of the information is contradictory[13,14]. In caesarean section the use of opiates does appear to reduce the incidence of recall[15,16].

It would probably be widely agreed that premedication can, in some circumstances, influence the incidence of awareness, but that this depends on dose, the drug used, and the time of administration. It would be unwise to rely on the use of premedication to ensure unconsciousness.

Volatile agents

All the evidence available points to the conclusion that using the volatile agents as adjuvants to nitrous oxide and oxygen reduces the incidence both of dreaming and awareness. Halothane appears to be effective[14,17] (see Table 22.1), as does enflurane[18].

Intravenous agents: droperidol

There is evidence that Innovar (a mixture of fentanyl and droperidol) reduces the incidence of dreaming[19]. It has also been found that the incidence of awareness was only 2% when opiates were used to supplement nitrous oxide (50%) in oxygen; this incidence is less than would be expected if nitrous oxide were to be supplemented in this concentration.

Technical factors

At induction

There is no doubt that some patients remember tracheal intubation, or the early stages of paralysis, when thiopentone is used for induction and the lungs are subsequently ventilated with oxygen[20,21]. On the other hand, in the author's unpublished series, mentioned above, no patient remembered the tracheal tube being passed, even though the dose of thiopentone never exceeded 350 mg (given rapidly): in these cases, however, the lungs were always and without delay inflated with nitrous oxide (70%) in oxygen prior to intubation, and not with oxygen alone. An adequate concentration of nitrous oxide must be built up before the action of the induction agent wears off.

The use of nitrous oxide in this way is, in practice, the most important factor in avoiding overt memory of tracheal intubation. However, it is not the only one: difficulty with passing the tube, prolonged attempts at intubation and too small a dose of induction agent are also important.

Another factor which may be of importance is the use of pulmonary ventilators with a large dead space. If this dead space has not been filled with anaesthetic gases, but with air or oxygen, there is a possibility that the patient may at least temporarily wake up when connection is made due to dilution of alveolar gas.

At the end of anaesthesia

The importance of this factor has been emphasized[22]. The main causes of difficulty are simply impatience on the anaesthetist's part and poor technique. The anaesthetist may reverse the action of a non-depolarizing relaxant too soon and may discontinue the administration of nitrous oxide too early and ventilate the patient's lungs with oxygen alone. The patient may complain of feeling the insertion of the last few stitches being inserted into the wound, may be aware of the tracheal tube's being in situ ('. . . a tube stuck in my throat which stopped me speaking') and of the suction of secretions from mouth, nose, pharynx and tube.

When very light anaesthesia is used, waking up at the end of anaesthesia is unpleasant. In the author's previously unpublished series, mentioned above, one patient in five found the experience of waking up very unpleasant – the worst part of the whole operation.

During maintenance of anaesthesia

Waters has given an excellent summary of the factors which may be operative during this period[23]. Failure of the nitrous oxide supply, usually due to the cylinder's having run out, is much less common since piped gases became the rule. The oxygen bypass is now spring-loaded so that if a finger is not kept on it turns off; previous designs of bypass allowed the oxygen to be accidentally knocked on and several cases of awareness have been recorded due to this factor.

Errors with pulmonary ventilators, however, still occur. Some ventilators driven by an electric motor can entrain air when used in open circuit mode if the gas supply is inadequate, and may entrain air in the closed system mode if there be a leak. Some ventilators with a 'negative phase' can suck in air and some ventilators will take in air if the ventilator is not attached to the gas supply.

It should be added that the present day practice of using a rather lower concentration of nitrous oxide than was usual previously, and using a volatile adjuvant as well, is not without its dangers. In these circumstances the vaporizer may run out and the anaesthetist not notice it. Several cases of awareness have resulted from this cause.

The patient

Little is known about why some individual patients should complain of being aware and others, subjected, it would seem, to a precisely similar technique of anaesthesia, should have remained completely narcotized. It could be expected that in a population the susceptibility to anaesthetic agents, if it were possible to measure it, would lie on a distribution curve but that other external factors might modify it.

Those who have a high intake of alcohol are more likely to be aware under anaesthesia[24,25]. This may apply to other central depressant drugs as well.

Special situations

Obstetric anaesthesia is a field of study in itself as far as awareness is concerned, though it has been suggested that the search for new methods of avoiding the difficulty has developed some of the features of an academic exercise. There are fortunately good accounts of the subject in text books on obstetric anaesthesia[26].

The difficulties of investigating paediatric patients are self-evident. There is evidence that paediatric patients can be aware[27], but there seems to be further scope for work in this field.

When thiopentone is used as the main agent for anaesthesia with relaxation provided by suxamethonium during bronchoscopy and laryngoscopy, there is, not surprisingly, a high incidence of awareness[28]; as yet, there are no completely satisfactory techniques for these procedures.

Avoidance of awareness

The use of very light anaesthesia with muscle relaxants is one of the great advances in the speciality. Patients still die from such avoidable factors as simple respiratory obstruction in the immediate post-operative period, and the only safe rule to follow is for the anaesthetist to leave the patient only when consciousness has returned and with it the ability to look after himself or herself in such simple matters as voiding vomit from the pharynx.

Even a patient who has suffered awareness would not be better dead. The appropriate question to be asked is not so much the simple one 'Can awareness be avoided?', but rather 'Can awareness be avoided and the advantages of light anaesthesia (in terms of rapid recovery of consciousness) still be retained?'.

This question does not require only a pharmacological approach. Impeccable technique, now less emphasized than it used to be, is also needed. For example, the patient may remember the passage of a tracheal tube if, say, after induction of anaesthesia with thiopentone, the lungs be inflated for a prolonged period with oxygen and nothing more.

In the present state of knowledge, the best pharmacological way of ensuring unconsciousness must be to supplement nitrous oxide with suitable, low concentrations of volatile agents delivered by an accurate vaporizer. All the evidence points to the view that volatile agents do indeed reduce the incidence of awareness and dreaming. They appear to provide the best and most flexible method of avoiding the incident.

Many anaesthetists rely on the use of opioids, such as fentanyl, in the belief that this will solve the problem. There is little direct evidence that this is correct, and good pharmacological reasons for supposing that it may not be.

In the first place the use of opioids does not necessarily involve smooth anaesthesia. But much more important is the fact that they do not, in themselves, produce anaesthesia save possibly in very large doses. They are drugs of great specificity which exert their action by attaching themselves to specific receptors. If they do reduce the incidence of awareness, they do so presumably by decreasing the arousing effect of nociceptive stimulation.

The evidence that the volatile agents reduce the incidence of both awareness and dreaming is better founded and the pharmacological basis more sure. They might genuinely be said to increase the depths of anaesthesia and, for this reason, might be considered, in a sense, as specific agents for this purpose. The appearance of these agents and of reasonably accurate vaporizers for them means that, when used in low concentrations, they provide the best and most flexible means of making sure that the patient is not aware; and in this way, they also enable the careful and skilled anaesthetist to guard against awareness as far as this is possible and at the same time retain the advantages of light anaesthesia.

References

1. CRILE, G. (1947) *An Autobiography*. Philadelphia: Lippincott
2. WINTERBOTTOM, E. H. (1950) Correspondence: Insuffucient anaesthesia. *British Medical Journal*, **1**, 247–248
3. HUTCHINSON, R. (1961) Awareness during surgery. A study of its incidence. *British Journal of Anaesthesia*, **33**, 463–469

4. UTTING, J. E. (1982) Awareness during surgical operations. In *Recent Advances in Anaesthesia and Analgesia*, 14th edn, edited by R. S. Atkinson and C. L. Hewer, pp. 105–119. Edinburgh: Churchill Livingstone

5. BEECHER, H. K. and TODD, D. P. (1984) A study of the deaths associated with anaesthesia and surgery based on a study of 599, 548 anesthesias in ten institutions 1948–51 inclusive. *Annals of Surgery*, **140**, 2–35

6. GRAY, T. C. and HALTON, J. (1946) Technique for the use of d-tubocurarine chloride with balanced anaesthesia. *British Medical Journal*, **2**, 293–294

7. GRAY, T. C. and REES, G. J. (1952) The role of apnoea in anaesthesia for major surgery. *British Medical Journal*, **2**, 891–892

8. MEYER, B. C. and BLACHER, R. S. (1961) A traumatic neurotic reaction induced by succinylcholine chloride. *New York State Journal of Medicine*, **61**, 1255–1261

9. BERGSTROM, H. and BERSTEIN, K. (1968) Psychic reactions after analgesia with nitrous oxide for caesarean section. *Lancet*, **ii**, 541–542

10. BLACHER, R. S. (1975) On awakening paralyzed during surgery. A syndrome of traumatic neurosis. *Journal of the American Medical Association*, **234**, 67–68

11. BRICE, D. D., HETHERINGTON, R. R. and UTTING, J. E. (1970) A simple study of awareness and dreaming during anaesthesia. *British Journal of Anaesthesia*, **42**, 535–542

12. CRAWFORD, J. S. (1971) Awareness during operative obstetrics under general anaesthesia. *British Journal of Anaesthetics*, **43**, 179–182

13. HARRIS, T. J. B., BRICE, D. D., HETHERINGTON, R. R. and UTTING, J. E. (1970) Dreaming associated with anaesthesia: the influence of morphine premedication and two volatile adjuvants. *British Journal of Anaesthesia*, **43**, 172–178

14. WILSON, S. L., VAUGHAN, R. W. and STEPHEN, C. R. (1975) Awareness, dreams, and hallucinations associated with general anesthesia. *Anesthesia and Analgesia*, **54**, 609–617

15. WILSON, J. and TURNER, D. J. (1969) Awareness during Caesarean section under general anaesthesia. *British Medical Journal*, **1**, 280–283

16. CRAWFORD, J. S., JAMES, F. M., DAVIES, P. and CRAWLEY, M. (1976) A further study of general anaesthesia for Caesarean section. *British Journal of Anaesthesia*, **48**, 661–666

17. MOIR, D. D. (1970) Anaesthesia for Caesarean section. An evaluation of a method using low concentrations of halothane and 50 per cent of oxygen. *British Journal of Anaesthesia*, **42**, 136–142

18. FARNSWORTH, G. M. (1978) Enflurane and the incidence of awareness in Caesarean section. *Anaesthesia*, **33**, 55

19. BROWNE, R. A. and CATTON, D. V. (1973) Awareness during anaesthesia: a comparison of anaesthesia with nitrous oxide–oxygen and nitrous oxide–oxygen with Innovar. *Canadian Anaesthetists' Society Journal*, **20**, 763–768

20. BOGETZ, M. S. and KATZ, J. A. (1984) Recall of surgery for major trauma. *Anesthesiology*, **61**, 6–9

21. McKENNA, T. and WILTON, T. N. P. (1973) Awareness during endotracheal intubation. *Anaesthesia*, **28**, 599–602

22. EISELE, V., WEINREICH, A. and BARTLE, S. (1976) Perioperative awareness and recall. *Anesthesia and Analgesia*, **55**, 513–518

23. WATERS, D. J. (1968) Factors causing awareness during surgery. *British Journal of Anaesthesia*, **40**, 259–264

24. TAMMISTO, T. and TAKKI, S. (1973) Nitrous oxide-oxygen-relaxant anaesthesia in alcoholics: a retrospective study. *Acta Anaesthesiologica Scandinavica Supplementum*, **53**, 68–75

25. TAMMISTO, T. and TIGERSTEDT, I. (1977) The need for halothane supplementation of $N_2O–O_2$–relaxant anaesthesia in chronic alcoholics. *Acta Anaesthesiologica Scandinavica*, **21**, 17–23

26. CRAWFORD, J. S. (1977) Obstetrics, analgesia and anaesthesia. *British Journal of Anaesthesia*, **49**, 19–23

27. McKIE, B. D. and THORP, E. A. (1973) Awareness and dreaming during anaesthesia in a paediatric hospital. *Anaesthesia and Intensive Care*, **1**, 407–414

28. BARR, A. M. and WONG, R. M. (1973) Awareness during general anaesthesia for bronchoscopy and laryngoscopy using the apnoeic oxygenation technique. *British Journal of Anaesthesia*, **45**, 894–900

Chapter 23

Final discussion and conclusions

M. D. Vickers

'Real' awareness

There must be few who would quarrel with the assertion that most serious cases of 'real' awareness have been associated with poor training, gross errors or accidents, or else dictated by special clinical circumstances. They could, therefore, have been prevented by better training or the use of currently available devices such as disconnection alarms, oxygen monitors and so on.

Once such cases are discounted, however, we are left with a residual problem of the occasional case of awareness when the anaesthetic technique has been apparently no different from that which has been successfully employed in many other patients without any such consequence. One explanation is that such a patient is at the extreme end of the distribution curve of minimum alveolar concentration (MAC) values in the population, or there may have been an undetected technical error.

Avoidance of 'real' awareness

No better explanation or hypothesis has so far emerged, but it should be possible to generate guidelines to minimize or even eliminate such occurrences, for example:

- Premedicate with sedative or amnesia-inducing drugs.
- Give more than a 'sleep' dose of induction agent if undertaking an immediate intubation under suxamethonium, particularly if using a short-acting induction agent.
- Do not totally paralyse the patient.
- Use adequate doses of analgesics: 'pure' analgesics may be less satisfactory from this point of view than those with euphoriant effects.
- Do not rely solely on nitrous oxide as the only inhalational agent to maintain unconsciousness when giving narcotics, unless there is a very good indication to do so.
- If supplementing with a volatile, maintain the end-tidal value of the volatile at least at 0.6 MAC when using 60% nitrous oxide or more.
- Monitor the composition of the fresh gas mixture.
- Always use a breathing system disconnection (low pressure) alarm, *which cannot be turned off*.
- Make sure that the inlet of fresh anaesthetic gases cannot be disconnected from a ventilator.

Reviewing the reported cases in the light of the above, the Medical Defence Union have been struck by the danger of relaxants with nitrous oxide and narcotic, unsupplemented by any volatile, in the hands of relatively inexperienced and unsupervised trainees. This seems to be a technique which should only be used by anaesthetists with quite a lot of experience.

It has to be recognized that these things could not be achieved overnight. End-tidal analysers for volatile agents, for example, are not cheap. It might take 2 or 3 years to achieve, but a strong recommendation now would help move things in the right direction.

'Hearing' under anaesthesia

What seems reasonably beyond doubt, however, to this author at least, is that surgical anaesthesia can *frequently* be associated with the capacity to detect and process auditory inputs. The consequences of this seem to be quite different, suggesting that the two phenomena may not be on a continuum. Auditory input is not the same thing as hearing. Patients who recall *hearing* things, recall more than the meaning of the words: they are spatially orientated, recognize accents etc. In short, they are *also* aware of having been conscious. This is very different from demonstrating, possibly by some indirect way, that the content or meaning of some auditory input has been retained. If these apparently different phenomena are really a continuum, the only safe solution would be to use sufficiently deep anaesthesia to abolish this capacity and this is apparently much deeper than that needed for most surgical purposes. The alternative is to use intravenous agents which disrupt the upper end of the auditory pathway at relatively non-toxic levels.

If, on the other hand, these two phenomena are not on a continuum, it has to be acknowledged that literally millions of patients have been in a state of being able to process auditory inputs; many presumably have done so, but apparently with little (or no) ill-effect. It is fairly important, therefore, to decide whether this negative observation is borne out by such scientific studies as have been conducted. The consensus of this book seems to be that auditory information is often processed if it is personally and psychologically disturbing and that it can then have long-term adverse effects. However, neutral material has not yet been shown to be in any way harmful, despite persuasive evidence of its retention.

The question then arises as to whether auditory inputs could be utilized beneficially, for example, to reduce post-operative pain. Some studies have attempted to show this but, in general, their methodology does not stand up to rigorous scrutiny. The use of patient controlled analgesia could provide an objective assessment of analgesic requirements in a double-blind study.

Dr Bennett (Chapter 15) reported some unpublished work on the incidence of the need for post-operative urinary catheterization (0/12 as opposed to 8/12 in the control group) in those given suitable suggestion under anaesthesia. He suggested that, contrary to natural expectation, smooth muscle function was particularly suggestible.

A note of caution should be registered, however, before anaesthetists are encouraged to behave as though the patient could hear everything. It would profoundly alter operating theatre behaviour and would soon leak out to the public at large. We have to be very sure of the lack of harm of this approach.

A further point to bear in mind is that patients emerging from anaesthesia are prone to hallucinate and everything that the patient 'recalls' may not be rooted in reality.

A consciousness monitor

Turning now to the situation in which light anaesthesia is desirable, what are the prospects for detecting incipient consciousness? The various parameters which have been described in this book really have been methods directed at measuring depth of anaesthesia: have any of them the potentiality for extrapolation back to detect the difference between consciousness and unconsciousness?

Of those considered, the tone of the frontalis muscle seems to be the only one which looks as though this is a real possibility. The seventh cranial nerve is primarily an autonomic nerve and the frontalis is almost a 'window' on the autonomic system. The 'tears of frustration', the frown of worry, the screwed up face of pain all register emotions which are not under conscious control. With the spectral edge of the EEG, or median frequency, or any other processed EEG signal there does not seem to be a clear cut-off, without overlap, between consciousness and unconsciousness. The other proposals (for example, oesophageal contractions) do not look at something going *into* the brain but at what is emerging *from* the brainstem. Switching on the halothane or other volatile largely gets rid of this problem, but unfortunately this approach cannot always be taken.

Testing a 'consciousness monitor'

The search for a monitor of consciousness raises questions to which it is not yet clear if there are answers. How would one recognize a false positive, i.e. the machine said the patient was awake but the patient did not subsequently think so? Would they have to be hypnotized? Remember: every false positive would result in anaesthesia being deepened for someone who apparently did not need it deepened.

Would a 5% false positive rate be acceptable?

When it comes to false negatives we need to be very much more stringent. The 'natural' incidence of awareness with current anaesthetic techniques is not known but perhaps 1% of caesarean sections would be a reasonable guess. Any equipment that failed to detect one in 10 of these would hardly be satisfactory. That would be a false negative rate of one in 1000 overall. This suggests that some 3900 caesarean section patients need to be subjected to investigation with no false negatives before confidence in the method could be felt. Quite a daunting prospect. It would be a virtually untestable instrument.

A higher probability of awareness could be deliberately engineered, for example, by having patients with the excluded limb able to squeeze in response to instructions. It would be interesting to see what an ethical committee would make of such a proposal.

Future research needs

One of the ironies of the developing situation is that the defence organizations are paying out sums in compensation for unintended consciousness, which greatly exceed the money that would be required to investigate the problem thoroughly. However, I doubt if that will encourage funding of the necessary research. Even so, several lines of research suggest themselves as urgently required. At very least there are promising experimental protocols for linguistic psychologists to explore what auditory information is processed and in what ways.

Of more practical value, several carefully controlled studies, not only double blind but tamper-proof, are called for: initially, to identify what kinds of auditory input (if any) are likely to be monitored by the patient and at what depth of anaesthesia; evidence of benefit of positive suggestions would be welcome; a comparison of inhalational anaesthesia and intravenous infusion anaesthesia is called for, to see if there are different effects on the auditory pathways.

Do different narcotic supplements have different effects? What level of dosage is necessary to abolish the phenomenon of auditory retention? Most of all, a major comparative study is needed of frontalis activity, the EEG, processed in various ways, auditory evoked potentials, meaningful auditory information, and occluded forearm in patients who have been kept 'light' under relaxants.

There may not be too many firm answers but plenty of new questions suggest themselves.

Patients' experiences of awareness during general anaesthesia

J. M. Evans

In order to obtain a useful sample of patients' experiences of recall during anaesthesia, an advertisement was placed in the personal columns of four national newspapers which traditionally carry such classified advertisements. It was hoped, by this means, to collect a sufficient number of patients from whom more could be learnt of their experiences and the effects it had upon them. It was not assumed that the sample collected by this means would be representative of all patients who had experienced awareness, but it was hoped that the sample would provide some useful additional information.

Advertisement

SURGERY Have you ever been conscious during a surgical operation when you were supposed to be anaesthetized? A medical research team would like an account of your experiences. Write in confidence. Box. No.

When replies to the advertisement had been collected and examined, a questionnaire and explanatory letter were sent to the patients which sought specific information and gave them the opportunity to provide free comment in addition to that already provided in their first reply – this was done in 1984.

Results

Thirty-three replies were generated by the advertisement from which 27 adequately documented cases were obtained.

The patients

The average age of the patients at the time of surgery was 35 years, ranging from 4 (two patients) to 54 years of age. A majority (70%) of the patients was female. Recollections were not confined to recent operations; recollection averaged 18 years with a range of 1–59 years ago.

The operation

The surgical procedures are listed in *Table A.1* by category associated with these cases of recall. One patient (No. 12) experienced recall on two separate occasions and thus 28 operations are listed. The nature of the sample does not allow any positive conclusions to be drawn about the frequency of awareness during different surgical operations; the presence of four obstetric operations is not surprising.

Table A.1 Surgical procedures by category associated with reports of awareness

Surgical procedure	Reports
General surgery	9
Gynaecology	6
Ear, nose and throat	5
Obstetric	4
Thoracic	3
Orthopaedic	1

The events recalled

Affirmative answers to the following specific questions were obtained from the questionnaire:

During the anaesthetic, did you experience any of the following?

Hear noises or recall conversation	85%
Feel pain	41%
Feel discomfort only	41%
Could you recall the position you were in?	96%
Did you experience fear or panic?	78%
Did you find yourself unable to move?	89%

Which parts of the operation do you think you recalled?

Beginning	41%
Middle	44%
End	30%

From a review of the free comment it was apparent that 33% of patients could recall sight also.

The post-operative period

In response to the question 'Did the events upset you?', 21 replied, 'yes'. No obvious feature of the patient or surgical procedure correlated with this response, but of the 21 patients who found the experience upsetting, 20 had experienced pain or discomfort, whereas only two out of the six patients who did not find the events upsetting had experienced pain or discomfort. Dreams related to the recalled events were experienced by 26% of the patients.

Two-thirds of the patients told the hospital staff of their experience, but only 30% talked to the anaesthetist about the events. Patients often expressed reluctance to discuss events with hospital staff for fear of disbelief or ridicule. The patients' general practitioner was told of the experiences by 22% of the patients. The usual response of hospital and medical staff appeared to be defensive, ranging from sympathy and a complete explanation at the one extreme to denial and amusement at the other. Many patients found the dismissive attitude of the medical staff a source of great annoyance and frustration. All of the patients eventually told a friend or relative of their experiences and this generated responses of disbelief, horror and sympathy. When asked to compare this experience with other unpleasant experiences in their lives, 41% of the patients considered the event to be the worst experience of their life.

Patients' comments

In their first reply and in the questionnaire, patients provided free comment and description of their experiences. Parts of their accounts (in order of receipt) which provide a fair description of their experiences, are abstracted below.

Patient 1   Male aged 54   Bronchoscopy (1978)

'The feeling of helplessness was terrifying. I tried to let the staff know I was conscious but I couldn't move even a finger nor eyelid. It was like being held in a vice and gradually I realized that I was in a situation from which there was no way out. I began to feel that breathing was impossible and I just resigned myself to dying.'

'Worse than being bombed and machine-gunned during the war – from the point of view of fear engendered.'

Patient 2   Female aged 29   Ectopic pregnancy (1977)

(Doctor's daughter)

'Thank you for giving me the opportunity to exorcise a haunting of many years. As soon as I was out of intensive care and able to feebly clutch a pencil, I scrawled down my experiences before it became distorted by memory, imagination and distance. I am confident that this account of surfacing during an operation is accurate because it is still etched upon my mind with terrifyingly vivid clarity. The consciousness was terrifying. PAIN. Christ, the pain! The desperate animal terror of trying to signal one's conscious state to someone, but unable even to twitch a bloody eyelash. This is a nightmare to end all nightmares, being horrifyingly unable to communicate anything because paralysed. (Curare?) Had as much vision as peeping through eyelashes when pretending to be asleep. Could see patent glazing of roof lights, huge circular lamps, recognized surgeon, houseman and senior registrar. 'Will you be playing golf this weekend, sir?' asked the senior registrar. Noncommittal grunt from sir. It's swabbing around the site of the wound that's pure torture. The pain then is so incredibly intense that you faint. I "fainted" several times, slipping back into black oblivion. Two years later, before going to theatre for an operation on the next (third) ectopic, I wept in terror at the thought of again coming round in mid surgery, but I didn't dare tell anyone in case they thought I was either lying or mad.'

'I wish now I had had the courage to talk to someone about it at the time, instead of sustaining the stiff-upper-lip "brave girl" nonsense.'

Patient 33   Female aged 26   Appendicectomy (1968)

(Nurse)

'I was given an intravenous injection in the anaesthetic room. I awoke in theatre whilst the operation was under way. I could hear voices talking casually whilst obviously "at work" – I then became aware that I was suffocating – although I could hear the voices I found I could not move an eyelid, finger or anything to indicate to them my desperate need for air. I could not shout or make a noise. I felt no pain. I remember no more but for a long time afterwards (especially whilst in hospital) I had to have a window open near me.'

Patient 4   Female aged 33   Ectopic pregnancy (1975)

'I had an experience which had troubled me for eight years and which has never been explained to my satisfaction. I was anaesthetized, at first quite successfully. I then began to recover consciousness and was aware of acute pain. I could also hear the conversation in the theatre and learnt that I had an ovarian cyst which was "palpable". I could open my eyes a little and see shadowy shapes around me. Because of the pain I tried to indicate that I was not wholly anaesthetized and had the nightmare sensation of trying to move a limb, without the power to do so. I struggled to make a sound and eventually heard someone say "Don't let her move her head". I think I was then put under a deeper anaesthetic.'

'The memory of the pain and my acute helplessness will always be with me. In a subsequent operation I was able to tell the anaesthetist who seemed to understand and assured me it would not happen again. It didn't, but what if I was unable to speak to an anaesthetist? I have wondered if I should wear some identifying disc or tatoo if I am liable to react in this way to certain anaesthetics.'

Patient 5   Male aged 50   Thoracotomy (1971)

'I felt my right arm was outstretched and I heard the surgeon say "Push his shoulder back" and I felt his spraying reaching the front of my chest. I panicked and tried to call out and was terrified that I would feel the surgeon's knife in my chest. I could not speak, I tried to open my eyes but could not, I managed to move my fingers and that was the last that I remember until I woke up in the ward.'

'I served in the Royal Navy in the Second World War and was in many campaigns, under fire by the enemy aircraft etc. . . . but it was not as frightening as my operation.'

'I am thankful to the surgeon, anaesthetist and the chest physician who arranged it all for me. I blame nobody for that awakening, it just happened.'

Patient 6   Female aged 24   Tonsillectomy (1935)

'I felt myself coming round but did not open my eyes but there was the feeling of a large spoon-shaped object gouging flesh from my throat and everything hazed over.'

Patient 7   Female aged 25   Casearean section (1957)

'I could hear the surgeon ask the anaesthetist whether I was sufficiently anaesthetized and the anaesthetist then lifted my eyelid and said I was. I saw there were several other people in theatre but I could not move or speak. I was terrified and tried to signal with my little finger. I was aware of an icy line being drawn on my stomach but I do not know whether this was antiseptic or an instrument being applied.'

'I only mentioned this experience to my husband some weeks later. I really doubted if he would believe, but he did and it was a great relief.'

'I have, ever since, had a horror of hospitals.'

Patient 8   Male aged 36   Skin graft (1976)

'The anaesthetic administered had a very nasty effect. In between what I can only describe as a horror show nightmare, I had periods of being awake, in which I saw the surgeons, their green theatre garb and the lights etc. I awoke in the recovery room feeling terrified. I later asked the name of the drug I had been given – it was apparently "ketamine", not normally used. It put me off hospitals for life. I always invent excuses not to go in for any suggested treatment.'

'The effect was so unexpected and lasted a good fortnight. The hospital doctors' attitude was the worst aspect, doctors sometimes appear very patronizing.'

Patient 9   Female aged 41   Hysterectomy (1975)

(Nurse)

'I would like to tell you of my unforgettable experience.'

'I came out of the anaesthetic as they were stitching me up – I felt acute *burning* pain every time the needle went in and could tell which type of stitching they were doing. I tried to move or yell, but couldn't flicker an eyelid. I could feel the warmth of the lights and hear the click of instruments and low voices and "canned" soft music.'

'I was simply terrified and thought I would probably die of "shock"; just as I felt I could stand no more I went under again.'

Patient 10   Female aged 36   Kidney operation (1983)

'During the operation I can remember coming round, I don't think I opened my eyes but I can recall the most excruciating pain in my left side, I was lying with my head lower than my body and on my right side. I can remember trying to scream but was unable because there was something in my mouth and throat.'

'I am still terrified in case I should ever need another operation of suffering pain to that extent and waking up while being operated upon.'

'How do I ensure that it will never happen to me again?'

Patient 11   Male aged 33   Thoracoplasty (1956)

'I soon realized that I was fully awake and could sense the ribs of my back being crunched painlessly. As my mind cleared I vividly remembered that I was lying on an operating table and I was undergoing surgery on the ribs of my back. I now heard remarks to the effect that I was awake. My energy in the days of post-operation was concentrated on regaining normality and I did not dwell on the above experience.'

Patient 12   Female   (a) aged 42 Hysterectomy (1960)
(b) aged 52 Appendicectomy (1970)

'This has happened to me twice. The first time at the start of a hysterectomy operation in 1960 and the second during a follow-up visit to the operating theatre after an appendix operation that went wrong in 1970. It has made me very nervous of an anaesthetic ever since.'

Patient 13   Female aged 21   Appendicectomy (1943)

'After some while I was taken into the operating theatre and laid on the table. I could feel the bright lights above me and thought any minute I am going to feel the knife. They took me back to the anaesthetic room for another injection . . . the operation went off successfully. It does not bother me, there was a war on and the hospital was being bombed at the time. I don't think it could happen these days but I am not afraid and always seem to resist the anaesthetic, fighting to stay awake.'

Patient 14   Female aged ?   Hysterectomy (?)

'I became aware of noises – machinery? – people discussing my "ugly mess", and somebody washing me from the waist down (open hysterectomy). Mentally *very* alert, I was totally paralysed. I could not open my eyes and when I tried to take a breath with which to speak I found I could not alter the rhythm of my breathing. I tried many times in panic but could not make a single physical movement.'

'When I repeated their conversation, no explanation was offered except to ask if I drink. I do not.'

'Two months later I was told I needed to have some bone taken from my hips to repair spinal damage (a double fusion) and I refused because of my previous experience.'

Patient 15   Female aged 7   Removal of TB glands in neck (1946)

(Doctor's daughter)

'Your advert rang many bells with me although the experience you talk of happened to me in 1946 at the age of seven.'

'I had been anaesthetized outside the theatre so when I woke up I saw two men in gowns and masks talking to the left of me in a room – pale green I think, and a large circle of light above me, I wondered where I was.'

'They continued with what they were doing and did not seem to notice "I was there". Subsequently I must have fallen asleep again.'

'The next day I saw the surgeon and told him what had happened and what they had been doing and saying – and he told me it was ridiculous, I could not have heard because I was asleep and neither could I have seen the inside of the theatre.'

'I wish that anaesthetists would admit it to patients that this *can* happen rather than dismissing it as nonsense. I felt far more distressed by the denial received from them. I had plenty of opportunity to discuss the subject with my father and his friends and colleagues. All, without exception, dismissed it as nonsense.'

'It was a totally real experience – and since I was a child nobody would believe what I was saying. I felt generally angry – particularly with the doctors. It has made me nervous about subsequent operations in case it should happen again – which it hasn't.'

'I should be very glad to know if this is a common occcurrence.'

Patient 16   Female aged 35   Caesarean section (1981)

'Throughout the operation I was aware of terrible pain – the anaesthetic was apparently sufficient to keep me from moving or giving any sign of consciousness but not to block any pain. I told my GP and also the doctor in the hospital. They just nodded but seemed not to take any notice.'

'I have tried very hard to put the whole experience out of my mind but although I have managed to put it to the back it is very difficult to forget such a nightmare horror.'

Patient 17   Female aged 36   Caesarean section (1968)

'The worst experience I have had. I would not have another baby. The only think I can imagine to be worse would be to be buried alive. I felt the cut and then a thud like an electric shock. This was repeated several times. I tried to sit up but could not move. I am due to go into hospital next week for another operation and I am still terrified. I had a hysterectomy four years later and I was hysterical in the small room next to the theatre. It took 45 minutes to try to calm me enough to get me into theatre. The nurse who came from the ward for me told me afterwards that I was clutching at things and refusing to leave the recovery room without my baby – so it looked as though I had been reliving my experience.'

Patient 18   Male aged 45   Hernia repair (1977)

'I came out of the anaesthesia and couldn't understand why I wasn't in the ward. I could see the surgeons at the end of the operating table and I thought "O my God, they're going to operate on me and I'm awake". I tried to tell them but couldn't speak – couldn't move. Then some logic took over and I thought "OK if I can't move and can't feel anything then I won't feel when they cut me". Then the surgeon told me what had happened. I shall never forget the experience and the memory of the theatre sister in her green uniform trying to reassure me will remain with me. It is probably the worst experience of my life. I was told later that I was allergic to the suxamethonium (a muscle relaxant) which had been given to me, and was unable to break it down.'

Patient 19   Female aged 28   Nose surgery (1970)

'I was given my anaesthetic injection expecting oblivion to follow. To my horror I did not go under immediately. I could hear very clearly and feel everything happening to me but I couldn't see and my eyes seemed to be closed. Also, of course, I could not move anything. I spent what seemed like a long time fighting to try to move something to tell "them" I was still awake. All this time the anaesthetist was trying to fit a metal object into my mouth, presumably for the airway, and cursing me because my jaw was an unusual shape and made it difficult to fit. Then followed a discussion on my jaw, nose and adenoids with the surgeon who proceeded to tell all the assembled about the horrors of the British National Health Service. It seemed a long time before I became unconscious.'

'The next day my surgeon wanted to dismiss it as a dream but he was amazed when I repeated the conversation word for word.'

'I am pleased to hear that research is being conducted on this subject. I hope it will enable other people to avoid having the same awful experience.'

Patient 20   Male aged 4   Tonsillectomy (1925)

'I woke up in the middle of a tonsil operation. I remember the scene vividly to this day; the surgeon was our family GP and I remember his face as it was then, not as it became in later years. I remember him reaching for the chloroform bottle and mask.'

Patient 21   Female aged 53   Colostomy (1976)

'During the operation I became conscious. I saw three men moving around me dressed in dark green overalls and wearing what appeared to be blue and white J-Cloths on their heads. One seemed to be pulling yards of tubing out of my mouth. I felt no pain and I heard a man's voice saying "Her eyes are open", and a different muffled voice saying "They shouldn't be open". I remember no more.'

Patient 22   Female aged 33   Caesarean section (1977)

'During a caesarean section I was fully conscious while I was being stitched up. The worst aspect of the experience was desperately wanting to move or speak and being unable to do so. Yet I could hear and see quite clearly, as well as feel pain.'

Patient 23   Male aged 4   Hernia repair (1944)

'I had such an experience forty years ago when I was four years of age. The experience imprinted itself on my mind and according to my parents changed my personality. The experience is still with me, in fact I think of it almost every day.'

Patient 24   Female aged 39   Laparoscopy (1982)

(Wife of Dental Surgeon)

'No loss of consciousness with first injection.'

'Paralysing injection administered – absolute agony in that arm. I screamed and thrashed about so they knew I was awake.'

'Paralysing injection works. Total alertness of brain and terror that they would start with me "still there". Totally unable to move.'

'Intubation felt – sensation but no pain.'

'I started praying as hard as I could (I am a Christian) and went unconscious immediately.'

'Exceptionally rapid mental recovery after operation. Of course I complained (informally) afterwards, so did my husband. Although I have made it perfectly plain that I was not going to sue anybody (I accept that mistakes do happen), nobody would admit that anything untoward had happened. Just an apology would have been nice.'

'The registrar was sent to see me the following day but would not admit anything. I am afraid I got angry and told him that if his Protection Society would not let him admit it to me, in spite of my undertaking not to follow it up, I hoped it would permit him to admit it to himself.'

'I have recently had another GA. Needless to say I was terrified. The senior consultant was the anaesthetist, the previous year's episode was accepted as fact and enormous care was taken to ensure that everything went smoothly. It did.'

Patient 25   Female aged 49   Hip surgery (1977)

'I was distinctly aware of the surgeon hammering the pin into my left leg, obviously I felt no pain and really didn't know whether I was conscious or unconscious. The following week I was to have a similar operation on my right femur and I advised the anaesthetist of my experience and asked to be put deeper under on this occcasion. I have no recollection of the second operation.'

Patient 26   Male aged 51   Sinus operation (1979)

'I told the surgeon the following day and his initial reaction was one of slight amusement tinged with disbelief. When I repeated word for word the conversation between him and the anaesthetist he was astounded.'

'I mentioned it to a friend at a dinner party some months later. It stuck in her mind so much that when she was the person who saw the advertisement she passed it to me.'

'I do not think enough care and consideration is given to the patient regarding the anaesthetic. To the professional staff it is just one more for the theatre and the highly emotional state of the patient is not noticed.'

Patient 27   Female aged 23   Appendicectomy (1963)

'I recall feeling the cut and the sensation of being "open" – the pain was awful – someone said "you are supposed to be asleep". Apparently I was "knocked out" again, as my next memory was waking in the ward.'

'None of the medical staff mentioned the incident. When I did, I was told "strange things happen during operations", meaning dreams etc. I still remember the incident vividly and used to dream regularly.'

'I have a very broad outlook on life – this experience is something I cannot push to the back of my mind and forget.'

Index